D0934684

HEALTH CARE AND EPIDEMIOLOGY

Health Care and Epidemiology

Edited by

WALTER W. HOLLAND and LUCIEN KARHAUSEN

with the assistance of ANGELA H. WAINWRIGHT

Sponsored by the Commission of the European Communities

G. K. HALL & CO.

MEDICAL PUBLICATIONS DIVISION

BOSTON, MASSACHUSETTS

Health Care and Epidemiology

Walter W. Holland and Lucien Karhausen, eds.

Copyright © 1979
G. K. Hall & Co.
Medical Publications Division
70 Lincoln Street
Boston, Massachusetts 02111

ISBN 0-8161-2176-1

79 80 81 82 83 / 5 4 3 2 1

Printed in Great Britain at the
University Press, Cambridge

Contents

Contributors

John Ashley, MB, ChB, FFCM
Senior Research Fellow and Honorary Senior Lecturer, Department of Community Health, London School of Hygiene and Tropical Medicine, Keppel Street, London WC1E 7HT, UK

Zbigniew Brzezinski, MD, DPH
Regional Officer for Epidemiology, World Health Organization Regional Office for Europe, 8 Scherfigsvej, DK-2100 Copenhagen, Denmark

Johannes Clemmesen, Dr med, med hc
Director of the Danish Cancer Registry and Department of Pathology, The Finsen Institute, Strandboulevarden 49, DK-2100, Copenhagen, Denmark

Maarten Hartgerink, MD
Director, Netherlands Institute for Preventive Health Care, Wassenaarseweg 56, Leiden, Postbus 124, The Netherlands

Ole Horwitz, MD
The Danish Institute for Clinical Epidemiology, 25 Svanemøllevej DK-2100 Copenhagen, Denmark

Johannes Ipsen, Dr med, MPH
Professor of Epidemiology and Medical Statistics, Socialmedicinsk Institute, Aarhus University, Vesterbro Torv 1–3, 8000 Aarhus C, Denmark

Leo A. Kaprio, MD
Regional Director, World Health Organization Regional Office for Europe, 8 Scherfigsvej, DK-2100 Copenhagen, Denmark

Ulrich Keil, Dr med, MPH
Post-doctoral Fellow, Occupational Health Studies Group, Department of Epidemiology, School of Public Health, University of North Carolina, Chapel Hill, N.C. 27514, USA

Michel F. Lechat, MD, Dr PH
Professor of Epidemiology, School of Public Health, University of Louvain, 1200 Brussels, Belgium

Geneviève Massé, MD, MSH (Harvard)
Professor, Department of Biostatistics and Public Health, École Nationale de Santé Publique, Avenue du Professeur Léon Bernard, 35043 Rennes-Cedex, France

Louis Massé, MD, DrPH
Professor, Department of Biostatistics and Public Health, École Nationale de Santé Publique, Avenue du Professeur Léon Bernard, 35043 Rennes-Cedex, France

André Meheus, MD, DPH
Lecturer in Epidemiology and Social Medicine, Faculty of Medicine, University of Antwerp, Universiteitsplein 1, Wilrijk B-2610, Belgium

Alessandro Menotti, MD, PhD
Assistant, Centre for Cardiovascular Diseases, St Camillo Hospital, Circ. Gianicolense 87, 00152, Rome, Italy

Donald Reid, MD, DSc, FRCP*
Late Professor of Epidemiology and Director of the Department of Epidemiology and Medical Statistics, London School of Hygiene and Tropical Medicine, Keppel Street, London WC1E 7HT, UK

Claude Rumeau-Rouquette, MD
Director of Epidemiological Studies in Mothers and Infants, Division of Medical-Social research, Institut National de la Santé de la Recherche Médicale, Chemin de Ronde, BP 34, 78110 Le Vesinet, France

Rodolfo Saracci, MD
Epidemiologist, Unit of Epidemiology and Biostatistics, International Agency for Research on Cancer, 150 Cours Albert-Thomas 69372, Lyon Cedex 2, France

Robert J. van Zonneveld, MD, PhD
Director, Bureau of the Council for Health Research TNO, Juliana van Stolberglaan 148, PO Box 297, The Hague-2076, The Netherlands

Jean Weddell, MD, FFCM
Senior Lecturer, Department of Community Medicine, St Thomas's Hospital and Medical School, London SE1 7EH, UK

* Sadly Donald Reid died during the preparation of this book

Introduction

Lucien Karhausen

A number of questions may arise in the minds of readers of this book, the first of which may well be: 'Why another book on health care?' The following may supply the answer.

Health care is the set of actions which aim at the improvement of individual and collective health levels. Whether medical care policies and procedures achieve their aims, and to what extent they achieve them, are questions of major importance to clinicians, epidemiologists, general medical scientists, administrators of medical care and health policy makers.

These questions are of particular relevance in the education and training of medical personnel and of planners for medical care. The growing importance of the field of health care assessment stems from the increasing complexity of modern medical science and from the great cost of medical care which is rising faster than the Gross National Product in most Western countries. Faced with this situation health economists are increasingly being asked to define priorities for medical care. Answers to these urgent questions about priorities cannot be left to economists or managers: medical scientists must be prepared to develop a useful dialogue with these disciplines and be able to propose appropriate measures and programmes to solve set problems. This book tries to define the methods which could and should be used at the interface between medical care policy makers and managers, and medical scientists.

The second question readers may ask is: 'Why another book on epidemiology?' The answer to this question must begin with agreement on what epidemiology is about. Epidemiology is one of the three basic tools of medical research. The first is clinical investigation which studies the disease process at the bedside or on pathological samples. It is focused on individuals and stems from the clinical approach based on the doctor-patient relationship. The second is experimental medicine which consists of animal research on disease models observed or experimentally produced in laboratory animals or on a particular biological system.

The third approach is epidemiology which is focused on populations. It uses statistical tools but differs from statistics in specific ways. It is often said that clinicians are interested in numerators, statisticians in denominators and epidemiologists in both. As a methodological approach, epidemiology exists throughout medicine and it has taken a prominent part in recent developments in medicine by becoming a kind of 'medical conscience' in its criticism of the conceptual apparatus, of the methods, of the aims of medicine and of the best ways to achieve these aims.

Epidemiology was initially defined by its objective which was the study of epidemics i.e. the disease processes which strike a large number of people at the same time in the same place. The word 'epidemic' is very old and was already in use in the Greek language ($\epsilon\pi\iota\delta\eta\mu oo$) unlike the word 'epidemiology' which was probably only first used in the second half of the nineteenth century.

It would be incorrect to confuse the history of epidemiology with that of the study of epidemics and infectious diseases. Johannes Ipsen, author of Chapter 3, often says that epidemiology is a science without content so that the definition cannot be improved by specifying the object of study: epidemiology encompasses the whole field of medicine. This broader concept of epidemiology has been included in various medical systems since Hippocrates' time. Environmental factors were stressed by the hippocratic school, and miasmas were fashionable in the Middle Ages. Internalisation of causative agents came of age with the advent of bacteriology and finally the developments of the last forty years brought the now generally accepted multifactorial explanation of diseases.

Various definitions of epidemiology have arisen only in recent years. They do not differ significantly from one another and they can be equally applied to the traditional study of infectious diseases and the new interest in non-communicable diseases. Epidemiology is generally defined as a discipline which studies the factors which determine the frequency and distribution of diseases and injuries in human populations. The International Epidemiological Association (Lowe and Kostrzewski 1974) prepared the following definition in collaboration with the World Health Organization (WHO): 'The study of the factors determining the frequency and distribution of diseases in human population'. Sartwell (1972) recalls that Alexander Gilliam once said that epidemiology is what an epidemiologist does. But what are epidemiologists actually doing?

It seems that an important aspect of what epidemiologists are actually doing, which is not covered by the above definition, is what Ryle (1936) called the natural history of diseases in his celebrated monograph. It is true that much of the epidemiological literature is concerned with the analysis of the facts which modify the course of diseases or the development of disabilities; and this is actually one of the main tasks of epidemiology. One could thus define epidemiology as the study of the factors determining the frequency, distribution or course of diseases, injuries, disabilities or other manifestations of a medical nature. This broader definition has the advantage of stressing not only time-, space- and person-related factors but also the disease process itself. Epidemiologists are interested in case-fatality rates, duration of diseases, and geographical variations of the appearance of diseases. Most current definitions tend to describe epidemiology as an activity which remains external to the course of diseases but this is contrary to the truth. Epidemiology plays a major role in the identification of syndromes and disease entities, in completing the clinical picture and in evaluating medical care. Therapeutic care is concerned with interventions by humans which alter in a positive direction the natural course of diseases (Cochrane 1972). Epidemiology is necessary to assess whether this actually happens and it is also concerned with the evaluation of preventive measures as well as of medical procedure in general.

The answer to the second question should by now be clear. Most existing texts present epidemiology as a medical discipline, external to the natural history of diseases, which is concerned with rates, high risk groups and explanatory factors which could lead to preventive measures. It is in fact just as concerned with studying and modifying the course of disease itself and this is why it plays a central role in development and evaluation of health care.

This book differs from most of the current texts by placing emphasis on this last aspect, which is so often neglected. It is therefore intended for epidemiologists as well as for public health administrators and health care planners and it should enable some sort of dialogue and exchange to develop between them.

It is sponsored by the Commission of the European Communities and is intended for use in the member countries both at a national and international level where it could act as a tool for collaboration and coordination.

Although the uses of this book may be wider ranging it concentrates on the evaluation of health care: concepts for evaluation of preventive, diagnostic, therapeutic and rehabilitative care have been developed and are widely used (Cochrane 1972). In particular they should be used to answer two major questions:

(1) Does the programme (services, treatment or rehabilitative regimen) give beneficial results, or more precisely, does the programme achieve the objectives stated before implementation i.e. altering the disease process in some way?

(2) What is the cost in terms of resources (money and manpower) and

of human suffering (by the patients or the general population) of achieving these objectives?

The first question is related to the concept of effectiveness. Effectiveness relates to the planned results and is defined as the extent to which the defined objectives are achieved. Efficiency, on the other hand, relates to the cost of achieving these objectives and it can be defined as the output or end result achieved in relation to cost in terms of resources, manpower or money.

Effectiveness can be assessed by controlled trials but the measure to be used must be determined beforehand i.e. before evaluation is done. The Veterans Administration Cooperative Study on Antihypertensive Agents (1970, 1972) consisted of a controlled trial of drug treatment of middle-aged male patients with mild or moderate hypertension. Various endpoints were used: mortality, morbidity (from cerebrovascular accidents, coronary heart disease, dissecting aneurysm etc.), systolic and diastolic blood pressure and electrocardiogram (ECG) tracing. From previous clinical trials it was expected that blood pressure would decrease. If however effectiveness is measured using stronger criteria, in terms of health effects (e.g. mortality, morbidity, ECG) it becomes more medically relevant. Hence this study showed evidence of benefit to the treated group when compared with controls. However the population studied was highly selected (i.e. middle-aged male war veterans, who had shown that they would take drugs regularly, and who had end-organ damage and a diastolic blood pressure above 115 mm Hg). In terms of health care, effectiveness implies that morbidity and mortality from strokes, coronary heart disease, hypertensive disease and cardiac failure will be decreased if all hypertensive patients in the general population are treated. The study does not show whether the same *level* of effectiveness should be assumed for the general population. In other words the fundamental question for policy makers remains unanswered: 'Is the systematic treatment of hypertensive patients effective?'

Effectiveness corresponds to evaluation of ultimate objectives of medical care i.e. the health benefits derived from any procedure. But evaluation of the accomplishments sometimes opposes evaluation of techniques (Hutchison 1967), of intermediate objectives or of the means by which ultimate objectives are reached. This last type of evaluation consists of determining whether a given preventive or therapeutic activity is being carried out according to predetermined standards which have been shown to be reasonably effective. Peer review systems such as the Professional Standard-Review Organization (PSRO) are of this type and consist of a programme of quality assurance based on the development of dynamic effective guidelines for efficiency which is defined as the skill with which resources (money, manpower, time etc.) are used to achieve a given end. Efficiency, like effectiveness, applies to diagnosis, prevention and therapeutic care: using effective methods inappropriately is inefficient, i.e. applying them at the wrong time in the wrong place and to the wrong people. An example of incorrect location was illustrated by Caplan (1964) who showed how brief active inpatient treatment for mentally ill patients was more efficient than outpatient care in the community.

The Commission of the European Economic Communities (EEC) commissioned the Panel of Epidemiology to prepare this book in order to help promote common research programmes; the book is the result of collaboration by some of the best epidemiologists from the member states. The primary responsibility for each chapter is recognized but in fact members of the Editorial Board and all authors contributed to the entire book by discussion, by offering suggestions for presentation and by some rewriting.

The Specialized Working Group of Epidemiology of the Committee of Medical Research of the EEC gave its full support to this undertaking and regarded it as an important step in the promotion of a coordinated medical care policy for Europe.

Moreover the Commission of the EEC, the Committee of Medical Research and Public Health of the European Community, and the European Office of the World Health Organization (WHO) recently decided it was essential to develop close links between the two organizations. The European Office for WHO will be engaged in the future in standardization of methods and terminology in medical research and in the evaluation of various systems of medical care, of health education, of screening procedures and of drugs. Dr Leo Kaprio, Director of the Regional Office, WHO Europe, was therefore invited to write a postscript and Zbigniew Brzezinski, WHO Europe Regional Officer for Epidemiology, collaborated in the final drafting of the manual.

REFERENCES

Caplan, G. (1964) *Principles of Preventive Psychiatry*. New York: Basic Books

Cochrane, A. L. (1972) *Effectiveness and Efficiency, Random Reflections on Health Services*. London: Nuffield Provincial Hospitals Trust

Hutchison, G. B. (1967) Evaluation of preventive measures. In *Preventive Medicine*. Clark, D. W. & MacMahon, B. (eds). Boston: Little, Brown

Lowe, C. R. & Kostrzewski, J. (1974) *Epidemiology: a Guide to Teaching Methods*. London: Oxford University Press

Ryle, J. (1936) *The Natural History of Disease*. Oxford: Oxford University Press

Sartwell, P. E. (1972) Trends in epidemiology. In *Trends in Epidemiology*. Stewart, G. (ed). Springfield, Illinois: Charles C. Thomas

Veterans Administration Cooperative Study (1970) Effects of treatment in hypertension. II. Results in patients with diastolic blood pressure averaging 90 through 114 mm Hg. *Journal of the American Medical Association*, *213*, 1143

Veterans Administration Cooperative Study (1972) Effects of treatment in hypertension. III. Influence of age, diastolic pressure and prior cardiovascular disease; further analysis of side effects. *Circulation*, *45*, 991

SECTION I

MEASUREMENT

The last method is an extension of the traditional practice of examining national or international differences in certain vital statistics for example infant mortality rates. A possible fifth area for study is the effectiveness of demand.

For the study of effectiveness Brotherston suggests: comparison of two contrasting systems of medical care and their effects on mortality; before and after studies to assess the impact of a new form of health care service; comparison of two similar populations experiencing different types of care (but opportunities to do this are rare); community surveys to assess patient satisfaction or attitudes to change; and the use of conditions which are modified only by medical treatment as 'indicators' of effectiveness.

The first three approaches to study of effectiveness are the most direct but the validity of findings is limited if changes in morbidity are affected by other factors unrelated to the amount and quality of care available. This potential source of error can be minimised in randomized controlled trials but such trials require full cooperation from clinicians and services concerned and there may well be ethical problems related to treatment of the conditions involved in such trials.

Effectiveness of demand is an important study area in order to answer the question: are those who are demanding a service demanding that which is most appropriate to their needs? And also: can the demand made be fulfilled by the available treatment or management methods?

There follows a general description of some of the underlying principles of observation which must be adhered to in any health care research.

CRITERIA FOR EPIDEMIOLOGICAL MEASUREMENT

All epidemiological measurements have to satisfy a number of strict criteria, some of which can be described in a few words but 'accuracy' warrants more detailed exposition.

Simplicity
Any test should be simple enough to be performed rapidly on large numbers.

Acceptability
A test must be accepted by most of the population under investigation, in general subjects should not have objections on ethical grounds or for reasons of increased risk.

Repeatability

This depends on variations by the observer, in the subject or in the method, it is only satisfied if the same observer obtains the same answer from the same subject at different times whatever the period in between, or if different observers obtain the same measure from the one individual.

Accuracy

To take account of the need for accuracy, one of the most difficult conditions to satisfy, requires the use of direct, that is *true*, measurement of the condition or symptom being investigated. Often this is not possible —instead a measure is taken of the best parameter available which is probably an indirect measure of the condition. An example is the frequency of symptoms such as cough or phlegm production which is accepted as an accurate measure of the prevalence of chronic bronchitis for a given population (examination of pathological specimens which would be the best parameter is rarely possible). Another example is blood pressure measurement: raised blood pressure is detected using an indirect measurement technique—a sphygmomanometer and cuff. The resulting measurements are no doubt highly correlated with the true intra-arterial blood pressure but there is no absolute one-to-one relationship. From such examples it is obvious that complete accuracy is neither possible nor essential for epidemiological study. It is sufficient that measurement is accurate enough to reveal differences which are unlikely to occur by chance.

It must also be remembered that measures may be either 'hard', that is they are physical measurements obtained with an instrument, or 'soft', that is subjective—as reported by a person. For example blood pressure, ventilatory function and visual acuity are 'hard' measures whereas symptoms of cough, chest pain, shortness of breath or feelings of depression are 'soft'—of course the labelling of something as a 'hard' or 'soft' measure is subjective in itself.

It must not be assumed that use of a complex (or even a simple) instrument to measure a given parameter will necessarily give an accurate reading. Instruments must be both properly calibrated and maintained and it must be remembered that people taking readings from such instruments are also likely to make errors or be subject to bias as are interviewers in the way they ask questions and interpret answers.

Sensitivity and specificity

In addition to the above criteria are the relative degrees of sensitivity or specificity: these will vary from test to test and from application to application and no test will ever be completely sensitive or specific. Specificity is defined as the number of individuals who are *not* affected by the condition in question and whose response to the test is negative, in relation to the number of unaffected individuals in the population. Sensitivity is defined as the number of individuals who *are* affected by the condition who *are* detected by the test in relation to the number of affected individuals in the population—they are both expressed as percentages. Table 1 illustrated the derivation of these criteria.

Table 1. *Fourfold classification of the concepts of sensitivity and specificity* (*Source: Cochrane and Holland 1971 and derived from Thorner and Remein 1961*)

Screening test results	Diagnosis		Total
	Diseased	Not diseased	
Positive	a	b	a+b
Negative	c	d	c+d
Total	a+c	b+d	a+b+c+d

a = diseased individuals detected by the test (true positives)
b = non-diseased individuals positive to the test (false positives)
c = diseased individuals not detected by the test (false negatives)
d = non-diseased individuals negative to the test (true negatives)

$$\text{Sensitivity} = \frac{a}{a+c} \times 100 \quad \text{Specificity} = \frac{d}{b+d} \times 100$$

The ultimate choice of a test may well depend on these two criteria, i.e. the relative cost of not detecting an individual who has the condition or wrongly diagnosing one who does not.

Reasonable cost

Although the term 'reasonable' is somewhat subjective epidemiological investigation must of course fit into an overall budget for health services taking into account the salaries and the time spent by individuals as well as the cost of materials and equipment.

From the criteria outlined above it can be seen that optimum conditions rarely apply: there is always some degree of error and to improve validity of findings this error must be recognised and estimated. The criteria involved in choosing a suitable study method include the particular condition, the method of treatment and linkage with future investigations; Cochrane and Holland (1971) have dealt with this in more detail.

STANDARDIZATION OF CLINICAL DIAGNOSIS

The equally vital criterion of standardized clinical diagnosis in epidemiological study is relevant in terms of all the criteria given above. Standardization should apply not only in clinical measurements of, say, blood pressure using a sphygmomanometer, but also in the estimates of the prevalence of, for example, articular rheumatism. In this context, a health care study would be necessary for the proper planning of physiotherapy services by ascertaining the actual morbidity for articular rheumatism by determining accurately its prevalence, both treated and untreated, in the community. A precise measure of prevalence and hence appropriate provision for need would depend on accurate diagnosis.

Clinical diagnosis in field studies depends on detection of a number of characteristic symptoms or signs that define the disorder in question. Determining the presence of a particular condition is subject to the vagaries of human response and habit in both the subject and the observer —recognition of this bias is as important as deciding on sample size and method of selection. Rose, Holland and Crowley (1964) described the observer and subject variation in measuring blood pressure; there is also evidence of an interaction between patient and doctor, for example when black patients have blood pressure measurements taken by white doctors (National Center for Health Statistics (1964) *Blood pressure in adults by race and area, United States 1960–1962, Vital and health statistics.* PHS Publ. No. 1000 Series 11 No 5. Washington: US Government Printing Office).

Error also occurs in the use of unstructured clinical interview where subjects react differently according to the format and structure of questions. Observers may vary in how completely they cover essential points, in the conventions they adopt to define diseases and the weight they place on specific items of history when deciding about the presence or absence of disease.

Observer variation may also occur in the use of structured questionnaires: Holland et al (1966) have shown the importance of assessing this variability. The United States National Health Survey (National Center for Health Statistics 1971) has described differences between various types of questionnaires—the differences in response when using questions which require definite positive or negative replies (closed questions), or those with more descriptive replies (open-ended questions)

Recent correspondence in the Lancet has highlighted the consequences of differences in definition for perinatal mortality which is often used as a measure of health care status in a particular area or a country. Goldstein and Butler (1977) point out that 'the international (World Health Organization) definition of perinatal mortality includes fetuses born without signs of life at or after 28 weeks from the date of a mother's last menstrual period, besides babies born alive at any gestational age who die within a week'. But they say that it is illogical to define a lower gestational truncation point for fetal deaths but not for live births although they realise that this is because of the legal requirement that all live births be registered and a cut-off point is necessary to avoid the difficulty of recording a large number of early deaths. They continue by saying that a common cut-off point for both live births and fetal deaths would have to be early enough to exclude a negligible number of live births but not so early as to include a large number of very early fetal deaths. Since some babies of under 28 weeks' gestation survive but few of less than 20 weeks' do it would be better to begin the perinatal period (both for definition of live births and for fetal deaths) nearer to 20 weeks.

Goldstein and Butler also point out that since a mother's recollection of her last menstrual period is often unreliable, birthweight rather than number of weeks might be a better way of defining the cut-off point for perinatal mortality. The International Conference for the Ninth Revision of the International Classification of Diseases (ICD) has recommended that: 'standard mortality statistics reported for purposes of international comparison should include only those babies born weighing at birth 1000 g or more'. Using data collected by the Ontario Mortality Committee, Goldstein and Butler have found a Perinatal Mortality Rate (PMR) of 22.8 per 1000 total births but with the proposed new definition the rate is 18.7 per 1000—an 18 per cent fall. They also point out that where countries have different average birthweights but similar distribution of gestational age there will be more babies under 1000 g in a country with lower birthweights and since there is a higher death rate among these babies use of the new definition will reduce PMR to a greater extent than in countries with higher birthweights.

They have examined babies of smokers and non-smokers during pregnancy. The latter weigh on average 170 g more at birth. Furthermore of babies born after 20 weeks of gestation to smokers 12.9 per 1000 had birthweights under 1000 g compared with only 6.3 per 1000 for non-smokers. PMRs for smokers were 25 per 1000 and for non-smokers 20.4 but under the new definition these figures would be 19.16 and 17.7 respectively: and so, a 23 per cent increase in perinatal mortality for babies of smokers becomes only 11 per cent using the new definition.

From their findings they conclude that despite the problems of using gestational age it is the only suitable method available.

In later correspondence Lewis and William (1977) cited work by Pharaoh (1976) who noted the differences between perinatal mortality definitions and statistics used in different countries: in France a baby born alive who dies before registration is separately recorded as 'died before registration'; in the United States the distinction between abortion and stillbirth is 20 weeks but 28 in most other countries, in Sweden the distinction is 35 cm physical length and 30 cm in Switzerland; the definition of 'signs of life' in an infant also vary.

Lewis and Williams (1977) have pointed out the difficulties of definitions when an arbitrary cut-off point is sought. They note that a universal definition of perinatal mortality would be valuable for comparisons between countries and provide valuable information for those who care for newborn and unborn infants.

Difficulties in standardization have led to development of standard clinical questionnairies for certain conditions where each question is precisely worded and asked in a fixed sequence. One such questionnaire was developed by the Royal College of General Practitioners in Britain (1961) for chronic bronchitis. It contained questions about the presence of respiratory symptoms—such as chronic cough, expectoration, breathlessness and wheezing. The items of clinical history were then grouped into syndromes of different severity which could be uniformly defined. A later version of this standard clinical questionnaire was adopted by the British Medical Research Council (Medical Research Council 1966) which recommended that the term 'chronic bronchitis' should be defined in terms of positive responses to specific questions on persistent cough, phlegm production and breathlessness on exertion. This questionnaire has been translated into all the Community languages (Van der Lende and Orie 1972).

Use of questionnaires in different languages does present problems because of the different emphasis a particular word might have. To achieve a foolproof translation certain steps must be taken: first the questionnaire should be translated into the second language by someone who is not only fluent in both languages but also an expert in the subject;

the questionnaire should then be translated back into the original language by another person with similar qualifications; at this point if there are variations it may be necessary to discuss the precise meaning of particular words or phrases.

Of course variations in the practical use of questionnaires not only depend on language differences but cultural differences as well, for example in the US or the UK. To check for these differences particular questions must be compared with an objective measure. It can be assumed that positive answers to questions on phlegm production are related to actual sputum production; subjects can be asked to collect sputum and the results can then be compared with their answers to questions. Alternatively if positive answers to questions about shortness of breath can be related to actual decrease in ventilatory function this provides a further check. If the relative differences in ventilatory function or sputum production for those answering the questions positively on phlegm production or shortness of breath and those answering the same questions negatively are the same in both countries it can be assumed that respondents in the two countries are interpreting the questions in much the same way.

The importance of diagnostic standardization in relation to the usefulness of results of health care surveys for international comparability, effective communications between research workers and productive collation of results has been stressed by Rose and Blackburn (1968). In their monograph of cardiovascular survey methods they related the recognized criteria for measurement to the various examination techniques in use for epidemiological investigation of ischaemic heart disease. Various annexes to the main text give examples of questionnaires which have been developed; for example, the London School of Hygiene Cardiovascular Questionnaire (Rose 1965), and questionnaires on dyspnoea, smoking and respiratory function. Examples of medical history forms are also given (US National Health Survey 1961). Bennett and Ritchie (1975) have produced a detailed guide to the design, use and evaluation of questionnaires including examples of different types of question.

Another example of standardization is in such techniques as x-ray and electrocardiograms. The Minnesota Code has been developed to improve the use of the latter (Rose and Blackburn 1968). The definition of characteristic signs on x-rays into uniform categories and supplemented by standard film of patients suffering from disease of differing severity has been used effectively in surveys of pneumoconiosis.

Unfortunately within the medical profession few diagnostic terms are used uniformly and there is also wide variation between doctors in interpretation of signs and symptoms (Raftery and Holland 1967; Fletcher 1952).

To obtain useful information it is necessary to obtain observations that are as homogeneous as possible. The International Classification of Diseases (ICD) can often be modified for use in general practice and in morbidity surveys but this type of classification requires individuals who are trained to use terms and examination techniques in a standardized way (Morrell, Gage and Robinson 1971).

In many circumstances sophisticated techniques have not been developed and many studies have to rely on more arbitrary methods of defining the presence of symptoms or conditions.

MEASUREMENT OF SERVICE USE

This is the second major function of health care studies. It is a complex subject because of the problems of inaccurate reporting and recording of simple events both by health service personnel, or service provider and the service user. As a result there are inaccuracies inherent in the regular statistical returns.

In his book *Health Care: Can there be equity?* which is a detailed study of health services in the United States, Sweden and England, Anderson (1972) describes the various measures of service use which can enable tentative comparisons to be made between countries. These include such figures as days spent in hospital, length of waiting lists, admissions, average length of stay, physician attendances and prescriptions filled. Of course the measurement will vary with the health service system in operation. More general demographic variables will also provide some measure of service use in a population, for example infant mortality rate, the age/sex distribution and mortality. All these specific and general variables can give some idea of whether the appropriate services are reaching the population that requires them and whether they are effective.

A specific example of evaluation of a service programme can be found in the WHO Report about a rehabilitative and preventive programme for patients who have suffered acute myocardial infarction (WHO 1973).

A number of studies with specific aims in the United Kingdom illustrate some of the problems involved in measuring the use of hospital services.

HOSPITAL SERVICES

1. *Complications following operation.* Holland, De Bono and Goldman (1964) found that only 70 per cent of complications following operation

were recorded and that recording was not affected by the severity of complications: hence, hospital records are inadequate for determining post-operative complications which might be a valid measure of the effectiveness of operative procedure. Holland, De Bono and Goldman also demonstrated the importance of using nurses' records, temperature charts and perhaps pathology reports to get full information.

2. *Laboratory investigations.* Whitehead (personal communication) in Birmingham, UK, found that between 20 and 30 per cent of laboratory investigations undertaken are never recorded on the hospital record because of difficulties in linking names and record numbers.

3. *Inpatient statistics.* Pearce (personal communication) at St Thomas' Hospital in London has recently attempted to check between two sources of inpatient statistics: the 'SH3'—an annual return of inpatient and outpatient data for every department in the hospital; and the Hospital Activity Analysis (HAA), data for which are collected for each patient and compiled by the Regional Health Authorities. Pearce found that the SH3 recorded 1500 patients treated in a given department over a year while the HAA had only 900 on record four months after the end of that year. Pearce's findings show that because of the time taken for patient information to be incorporated in the HAA it is not an accurate research tool for short-term use.

4. *Patient selection.* Bennett (1966) showed, by means of an analysis of cases treated in a London teaching hospital, that there is considerable selection of patients by diagnostic categories and age groups. In this particular analysis it was found that, in relation to the distribution of various conditions in the hospital catchment area, there was an excess of cases of certain specialist categories but a smaller case load from respiratory disease and injuries; this apparently reflected clinical research interests. A tendency to concentrate on the 15–64 age group in both sexes was also noted.

5. *Data sources.* Clarke and Bennett (1971) in a study of an urban and a rural area showed some of the problems of measurement of hospital use from hospital activity data, in recording of referrals by general practitioners and by interview of a random sample of the catchment area population. The need to use more than one source of data to gain an accurate picture was illustrated.

6. *Service-user information versus hospital records.* Palmer (1969) undertook a study to compare reports of attendance as outpatients or inpatients with hospital records at a number of London hospitals. Service-user information was collected by asking respondents if they had used a particular service, this is a technique used in most household surveys

such as the United States Health Interview Survey. Palmer et al used a six-month recall period (most such studies use a two-week recall) for events resulting in attendance at hospital including admission, and this was found to be reasonably accurate. It was found that older people and members of lower social classes were less likely to have accurate recall of events. These findings illustrate the importance of recognizing possible sources of error in reported information.

GENERAL PRACTITIONER SERVICES

Because the need for general practitioner services is dictated by morbidity experienced in the population it is a measure of morbidity which can provide a useful indicator for service provision.

The French household survey of 1970 collected information from 7400 households about illness and disability, medical products and services used, the reasons for their use, number of days spent in bed and interruption of normal activity as well as about demographic, social and economic factors which might influence morbidity (Mizrahi and Mizrahi 1977). These authors describe how bias was introduced by a lower response rate to the survey in Paris than in the provinces and there was also over-representation of children and fewer men in the 20–29 years age group. They also note the reluctance of people to disclose information about alcoholism or mental illness in the family which is yet another source of bias.

In Finland between 1964 and 1968 a similar household survey took place (Purola et al 1968). It had the specific objective of describing the level of service use in different parts of the country and in different population groups before introduction of a sickness insurance scheme. Particular attention was paid to sickness expenditure in families, and the effects of social conditions on service use, for example the degree of urbanization. Such household interview surveys have been shown to provide essential information particularly for accurate estimation of, for example, days of confinement to bed, acute mild sickness or injury which does not lead to physician attendance, or phenomena resulting from illness such as sickness absence. The use of interviews is also particularly relevant for relating service use to demographic, social and economic factors.

Morrell (1971) has developed techniques to assess the demand for general practitioner services in the UK. He performed an analysis of the age, sex and social class structure of a population consulting three doctors in an area of London and related it to presenting symptoms and principal diagnoses. A number of computer checking methods were used to measure the various errors in recording. It was found that the following population groups made a greater demand on health services: women; the elderly and young children; and members of social class III compared with IV and V, and I and II. A further finding was that respiratory diseases accounted for 25 per cent of all consultations and mental illness for 12 per cent. A pattern of the likely demand for general practitioner services for this particular area can thus be established and perhaps used to adjust service provision where necessary.

Surveys like those performed in Finland and France are described in more detail in *National Health Surveys in the European Economic Community* (Armitage 1977). Various surveys and the resulting health information systems are described for all the EEC countries and the US together with papers about health indicators, uses of national survey systems in epidemiological research and the economic aspects of health information.

The above examples illustrate that great care must be taken in assessing accuracy of recording of events by service providers and users as well as in recording of symptoms and physiological measurements. It should not be assumed that statistics gathered from hospital or GP records are an accurate picture of the use of health services.

CONCLUSION

A number of recent publications are worth mentioning because they illustrate how measurements of morbidity and service use are made and also how some such measures can be of use in allocation of resources. The need for fair allocation of resources has been realised particularly where funds are limited but even where they are not most people would approve the doctrine of equal accessibility to equal resources.

Measurement in health services has become a vital prerequisite for establishing norms, level and quality of service provision. In the past such measurement has concentrated largely on the *process* of providing care but now with restraint imposed by ever increasing costs standards of *outcome* should be emphasised. McLachlan (1976) has pointed out the inadequacy of many of the methods available.

A two volume publication entitled *Quality of Medical Care Assessment Using Outcome Measures*[1] (Brook et al 1977; Avery et al 1977) describes an attempt to develop specific short-term outcome measures for medical

[1] A summary of these reports can be obtained from the National Center for Health Services Research, Office of Scientific and Technical Information, 3700 East-West Highway, room 7-44, Hyatsville MD 20782, USA.

and surgical care given to patients with one of eight conditions including breast cancer, tonsillectomy and ischaemic heart disease. Nursing homes and a chronic disease hospital have provided the location for a detailed study into development of outcome measures in long-term care for chronic conditions (Jones, Densen and McNitt 1977).

One particular example of measurement in use for allocating resources is the result of work done by the Resource Allocation Working Party in the UK (Department of Health and Social Security 1976). This describes objective measurable criteria, for example age/sex standardized mortality ratios for different parts of the country and illustrates how these can be used to distribute revenue and capital resources to the 14 National Health Service Regions. This method of distribution has replaced other more subjective methods whereby money was allocated on the basis of the previous year's expenditure plus an allowance for inflation: such methods could not fail to perpetuate inequalities—partly created by individual advocacy.

Health Care: an International Study (Kohn and White 1976) describes a worldwide health survey which attempted to compare morbidity and service use between a number of countries. Immense differences between countries, however, in service use and symptom reporting precludes this study for use in decisions on resource allocation since no account was taken of such differences in calculation. From the data presented it is also difficult to distinguish between the effect of service supply or reported morbidity level and on use of services. The book does provide useful details of methods of morbidity measurement and service use including questionnaires, fieldwork procedures and data processing.

It is apparent that further work is needed to develop outcome measures to, for example, assess changes in mortality from a given condition, functional ability in sufferers from long-term conditions and satisfaction with services. In any of this work in future the principles of epidemiological investigations outlined in this chapter must be adhered to.

The following chapters will describe current epidemiological techniques for measurement purposes. The many examples given illustrate some problems inherent in this type of research and they will also give useful guidance to those who intend to embark on such studies.

REFERENCES

Anderson, O. W. (1972) *Health Care: Can there be Equity?* The United States, Sweden and England. New York: John Wiley

Armitage, P. (1977) *National Health Survey Systems in the European Economic Community.* Proceedings of a conference held in Brussels on 6–8 October 1975, Commission of the European Communities

Avery, A. D., Lelah, T., Solomon, N. E., Harris, L. J., Brook, R. H., Greenfield, S., Ware, J. E. Jr. & Avery, C. H. (1977) *Quality of Medical Care Assessment Using Outcome Measures: Eight Disease-Specific Applications.* (Obtainable from National Technical Information Service, Springfield VA, 22161, USA)

Bennett, A. E. (1966) Case selection in a London teaching hospital. *Medical Care, 4,* 138

Bennett, A. E. & Ritchie, K. (1975) *Questionnnaires in Medicine. A Guide to their Design and Use.* London: Oxford University Press for the Nuffield Provincial Hospitals Trust

Brook, R. H., Avery, A. D., Greenfield, S., Harris, L. J., Lelah, T., Solomon, N. E. & Ware, J. E. Jr. (1977) *Quality of Medical Care Assessment Using Outcome Measures: an Overview of the Method.* Supplement to *Medical Care,* 15 (9) (Obtainable from National Technical Information Service, Springfield VA, 22161, USA)

Brotherston, J. (1962) Medical care investigation in the health service. In *Towards a Measure of Medical Care.* London: Oxford University Press for the Nuffield Provincial Hospitals Trust

Clarke, M. & Bennett, A. E. (1971) Problems in the measurement of hospital utilization. *Proceedings of the Royal Society of Medicine, 64,* 795

Cochran, W. G. (1953) *Sampling Techniques.* New York: Wiley Publications in Statistics

Cochrane, A. L. & Holland, W. W. (1971) Validation of screening procedures. *British Medical Bulletin, 27*

Cooper, B. & Morgan, H. G. (1973) *Epidemiological Psychiatry.* Springfield, Illinois: Charles C. Thomas

Fletcher, C. M. (1952) The clinical diagnosis of pulmonary emphysema —an experimental study. *Proceedings of the Royal Society of Medicine, 45,* 577

Goldstein, H. & Butler, N. (1977) Definition of perinatal mortality (letter). *Lancet, 1,* 1254

Department of Health and Social Security (1976) *Sharing Resources for Health in England.* Report of the Resource Allocation Working Party. London: Her Majesty's Stationery Office

Holland, W. W. (1977) A general view. In *Epidemiology and Health.* Holland, W. W. & Gilderdale, S. (eds). London: Henry Kimpton

Holland, W. W., Ashford, J. R., Colley, J. R. T., Morgan, D. C. & Pearson, N. J. (1966) A comparison of two respiratory symptoms questionnaires. *British Journal of Preventive and Social Medicine, 20,* 76

Holland, W. W., De Bono, E. & Goldman, A. J. (1964) Inpatient records: an investigation of their content and handling at St Thomas' Hospital. *Lancet*, *1*, 819

Jones, E. W., Densen, P. M. & McNitt, B. J. (1977) *An Approach to the Assessment of Long-term Care*. Executive Summary. Boston: Harvard Center for Community Health and Medical Care

Kish, L. (1967) *Survey Sampling*. New York: John Wiley

Kohn, R. & White, K. L. (1976) *Health Care: An International Study*. London: Oxford University Press

Lewis, D. M. & Williams, G. F. (1977) Definition of perinatal mortality (letter). *Lancet*, *2*, 86.

McLachlan, G. (1976) *A Question of Quality?* London: Oxford University Press for the Nuffield Provincial Hospitals Trust

Medical Research Council (1965) Definition and classification of chronic bronchitis for clinical and epidemiological purposes. A report to the MRC by their Committee on the Aetiology of Chronic Bronchitis. *Lancet*, *1*, 775

Mizrahi, A. & Mizrahi, A. (1977) Assessing the morbidity of the population on the basis of household surveys. In *National Health Survey Systems in the European Economic Community*. Proceedings of a conference held in Brussels on 6–8 October 1975. Armitage, P. (ed). Luxembourg: Commission of the European Communities

Morrell, D. C., Gage, H. G. & Robinson, N. A. (1971) Patterns of demand in general practice. *Journal of the Royal College of General Practitioners*, *19*, 331

Moser, C. A. & Kalton, G. (1971) *Survey Methods in Social Investigation*. London: Heinemann

National Center for Health Statistics (1971) Effect of some experimental techniques for reporting in the Health Interview Survey. *Vital and Health Statistics*. PHS Publication No. 1000, Series 2, No. 41. Public Health Service, Washington, US Governmental Printing Office

Palmer, J. W., Kasap, H. S., Bennett, A. E. & Holland, W. W. (1969) The use of hospitals by a defined population. A community and hospital study in North Lambeth. *British Journal of Preventive and Social Medicine*, *23*, 91

Pharaoh, P. O. D. (1976) International comparisons of perinatal and infant mortality rates. *Proceedings of the Royal Society of Medicine*, *69*, 335

Purola, T., Kalimo, E., Sievers, K. & Nyman, K. (1968) *The Utilization of Medical Services and its Relationship to Morbidity, Health Resources and Social Factors*. Helsinki: Research Institute for Social Security

Raftery, E. B. & Holland, W. W. (1967) Examination of the heart: an investigation into variation. *American Journal of Epidemiology*, *85*, 438

Rose, G. (1965) Standardisation of observers in blood-pressure measurement. *Lancet*, *1*, 673

Rose, G. A. & Blackburn, H. (1968) *Cardiovascular Survey Methods.* WHO Monograph Series No. 56, Geneva: World Health Organization

Rose, G. A., Holland, W. W. & Crowley, E. A. (1964) A sphygmomanometer for epidemiologists. *Lancet, 1,* 296

Rosen, G. (1972) The evolution of social medicine. In *Handbook of Medical Sociology,* 2nd Ed. Freeman, H. E., Levine, S. & Reeder, L. G. (eds). New Jersey: Prentice Hall

Royal College of General Practitioners (1961) Chronic bronchitis in Great Britain. *British Medical Journal, 2,* 973

Stuart, A. (1968) *Basic Ideas of Scientific Sampling.* No. 4 in Griffin's Statistical Monographs and Courses. London: Charles Griffin

Tyrell, M. (1975) *Using Numbers for Effective Health Service Management.* London: William Heinemann Medical Books

Van der Lende, R. & Orie, N. G. M. (1972) The MRC-ECCS Questionnaire on respiratory symptoms (Use in Epidemiology). *Scandinavian Journal of Respiratory Diseases, 53,* 218

Woodham-Smith, C. (1951) *Florence Nightingale 1820–1910.* London: Penguin

White, K. L. & Henderson, M. M. (1976) *Epidemiology as a Fundamental Science.* New York: Oxford University Press

World Health Organization (1966) *Sampling Methods in Morbidity Surveys and Public Health Investigations.* WHO Expert Committee on Health Statistics Technical Report No. 36

World Health Organization (1973) *Evaluation of Comprehensive Rehabilitative and Preventive Programmes for Patients after Acute Myocardial Infarction.* Report of two Working Groups—Prague 4–7 October 1971, Moscow 27–30 November 1972. Copenhagen: WHO Regional Office for Europe

SUGGESTED TEXTS FOR BACKGROUND READING

Abramson, J. H. (1976) *Survey Methods in Community Medicine.* Edinburgh: Churchill Livingstone

Alderson, M. (1976) *An Introduction to Epidemiology.* London: Macmillan

Holland, W. W. (1970). *Data Handling in Epidemiology.* London: Oxford University Press

Holland, W. W. & Gilderdale, S. (1977). *Epidemiology and Health.* London: Henry Kimpton

Lilienfeld, A. M. (1976) *Foundations of Epidemiology.* New York: Oxford University Press

Reid, D. D. (1960) *Epidemiological Methods in the Study of Mental Disorders.* Public Health Papers 2. Geneva: World Health Organization

CHAPTER 2

Implications of Measurement

Zbigniew Brzezinski

The main problem areas in which health measurements are needed most are briefly described. These include identification of major health problems, setting priorities, formulating goals and objectives of health programmes, allocation of resources, selection of strategies for delivery of services, and evaluation of health programmes and services. Several examples on utilization of health measurements in the process of planning and administration of health services are given. Some problem areas in which there is a need for further research and development of operationally feasible health measurements are identified.

The development of health services and the improvement of health care have been influenced by tradition, culture, the state of medical knowledge and technology, economy, ideology and politics; the relative importance of each has varied from country to country and from one historical period to another. However, not until recently, has the need emerged to base the development of health care on a rational, comprehensive and systematic approach. Mahler (1975), while discussing the dilemma of contemporary health care, formulated the following four questions faced by anyone responsible for decision making on health matters:

'1. Is it possible to assign health resources within a country on a problem-solving basis (using different mixes of preventive, curative, promotive and rehabilitative action)?

'2. What medical interventions are truly effective and specific for prevention, treatment, or rehabilitation, as measured in objective terms?

'3. Can such medical interventions and the risk groups to which they should be applied be described objectively and in such a manner that the amount of skill and knowledge required for their application can be assessed?

'4. Is it possible to design a health care establishment to carry out the above tasks which will result in the most meaningful interventions reaching the greatest proportion of persons at risk, as early as possible, at the least cost, and in an acceptable manner?'

To obtain answers to these questions, which provide the rational basis for health policy making and developing health care services, epidemiological research should not only be intensified but enlarged in scope beyond the traditional boundaries. This implies more involvement of epidemiology and epidemiologists in planning, programming, management and evaluation of health services and health promoting activities (Holland and Gilderdale 1977). The availability of proper and operationally feasible measurements is of primary importance for any of these processes (WHO 1978).

The question of how such measurements are being developed and used in various kinds of epidemiological studies is dealt with throughout this book. Here, it is intended to point out some of the main problem areas in which the health measurements are needed most.

The first and fundamental issue is the identification of major health problems and health needs in a population and if possible estimation of future service needs. The health measurements in this context are used for decisions related to setting health priorities and formulating goals, objectives and health programme targets either at a national (Lalonde 1974) or an international level (WHO 1976a).

In view of the rising costs of health care on one hand and the growing health needs and demand for health services on the other, the attainment of specific targets and objectives requires proper allocation of resources and selection of appropriate strategies for the delivery of services. Both problems call for suitable measures to support decision making: recently an interesting solution to the first was developed in the United Kingdom by the Resource Allocation Working Party (DHSS 1976) and resulted in an important change in budget allocation methods.

The second problem is more complex. The impact of any system of health care is so dependent on the conditions of physical and social environment in a given population that no universal solution can be offered: a suitable approach must be sought taking into account all local circumstances: A very useful example is provided by a joint UNICEF/ WHO study (Djukanovic and Mach 1975) the starting point for which was the failure of conventional health services and approaches to make any appreciable impact on health in developing populations.

In addition to the above-mentioned decisions of a general strategic character, the planning process involves tactical and operational considerations which also require suitable measurements in order to assess

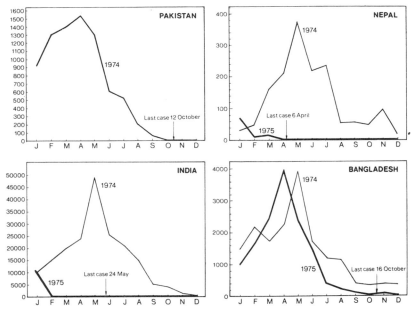

Figure 1. Smallpox cases in four Asian countries 1974–1975, showing date of onset of rash for the last known case in each country (Source: WHO Chronicle, 1976, vol. 30, 4)

equity, coverage, appropriateness, accessibility, availability, efficacy, efficiency, effectiveness and utilization of the planned services (Anderson 1977).

Apart from planning, such measurements are essential for implementation and management of health programmes and services. At each stage of implementation, it is necessary to measure how the programme or service is functioning and to assess if it is producing the required results. This kind of monitoring is required in both new and existing, ongoing programmes and services. The measurements involved are of input, process and outcome of health care.

Although all three types of measurement are needed for management, measures of outcome are particularly important. It is not enough to know what resources are committed and what kind of services are provided; and neither is it enough to measure how the available services are being used (Kohn and White 1976) unless the resulting health benefits to the patient and community can be shown. This task is relatively easy when the health benefit is apparent from the problem reduction in terms of cases of a disease, for example, tuberculosis (Härö 1976) or smallpox (Figure 1), but it is much more difficult in chronic or long-term conditions (Densen 1976). This is one of the problem areas in which further research is much needed.

The outcome measurements relate closely to the broader problems of evaluation of health programmes and services, and of evaluative research. In principle, evaluation is incorporated in the planning and managing processes and implies the identification of objectives and the asessment of how and to what extent these objectives have been achieved (WHO 1976b). However, in spite of a need for evaluation of all measures used in health programmes and services, there are few published examples of evaluation of more comprehensive programmes or systems of services, and only occasionally by evaluative surveys (Purola, Kalimo and Nyman 1974).

There are other problem areas like basic research on disease causation and natural history, and epidemiological surveillance: these however, are the traditional fields of epidemiology with well-established reputations. It is sufficient to mention here that the results of these investigations are also of importance for health planners and administrators, since they provide fundamental knowledge for planning of any health intervention, programme and service.

REFERENCES

Anderson, D. O. (1977) Priorities and planning. In *Epidemiology and Health*. Holland, W. W. & Gilderdale, S. (eds). London: Henry Kimpton

Densen, P. M. (1976) Epidemiologic contributions to health services research. *American Journal of Epidemiology*, *104*, 478

Department of Health and Social Security (1976) *Sharing Resources for Health in England*. Report of the Resource Allocation Working Party. London: Her Majesty's Stationery Office

Djukanovic, V. & Mach, E. P. (1975) *Alternative Approaches to Meeting Basic Health Needs in Developing Countries*. Geneva: World Health Organization

Holland, W. W. & Gilderdale, S. (1977) *Epidemiology and Health*. London: Henry Kimpton

Härö, A. S. (1976) Anti-tuberculosis programmes in Finland: Evaluation of current activities. *Tuberculosis and Respiratory Diseases Yearbook*, *5* (May)

Kohn, R. & White, K. L. (1976) *Health Care: An International Study*. London: Oxford University Press

Lalonde, M. (1974) *A New Perspective on the Health of Canadians.* Ottawa: Government of Canada

Mahler, H. (1975) Health—a demystification of medical technology. *Lancet, 2,* 829

Purola, T., Kalimo, E. & Nyman, K. (1974) *Health Services Use and Health Status under National Sickness Insurance: an Evaluative Resurvey of Finland.* Helsinki Research Institute for Social Security

WHO (1976a) *Sixth General Programme of Work Covering a Specific Period 1978–1983 Inclusive.* Geneva: World Health Organization

WHO (1976b) *Randomised Trials in Preventive Medicine and Health Service Research: Report on a Study Group.* Copenhagen: WHO Regional Office for Europe

WHO (1978) *Measurement of Levels of Health.* Copenhagen: WHO Regional Office for Europe (In press)

SECTION 2

HEALTH STATISTICS

CHAPTER 3

Use of Vital Statistics

Johannes Ipsen

Of the several population counts that constitute vital statistics, births and deaths are mainly discussed in this chapter. Births are used as numerators in population growth measurements, and as denominators in measures of deaths and defects, perinatally and in the first 12 months of life. Births are proportionately grouped by obstetric, physiological and socioeconomic attributes.

Deaths are discussed in terms of general and cause-specific mortality, and in relation to age, sex and social and demographic characteristics of the population. Methods for obtaining age standardized expressions for mortality of specified groups of persons, for example Standard Mortality Ratio, are described and their advantages and disadvantages mentioned.

Classification by cause of death through international systems is described. The uses of proportional and population-based mortality conclude the chapter.

INTRODUCTION

Births and deaths are the two basic events that are compiled into annual vital statistics for a given population and changes in these 'measures' constitute the principal indicators of growth and decline of a nation or community. Apart from, in very rare circumstances, other events, such as migration, have an insignificant effect on the existing population and its size. However, several communities have experienced temporary population changes as a result of migration or expansion of particular administrative areas. Any reader who is familiar with national or local history will probably know some good examples.

This chapter is concerned with measures of births and deaths, as they are used in epidemiological studies of causes of ill-health, evaluation of needs for health care, and assessment of effectiveness of prevention and cure. The basic data, i.e. official counts, are shared by demographers and epidemiologists, but the various users put differing emphasis on the subgrouping of vital statistics tables offered in official publications.

Vital statistics are historically produced for purely political purposes, the word 'statistics' is actually derived from 'state'. The usefulness of vital records, i.e. listing of events, births and deaths, is dependent on how much detail is collected in terms of personal attributes, places and times, on the accuracy of the recording, and lastly on the delay before official statistics are published.

While the absolute numbers of births and deaths are particularly important for demographic analysis and prediction, epidemiological analysis has two different uses for these data. First, in considering all the events in the population of a given area and the relevant time trends, epidemiologists will focus on the determinants of health and illness in assessing population decrease and growth, while the influence of political, economic, and social aspects might be towards demographic studies. The trend is fortunately towards a closer integration of the two scientific endeavours.

More often the use of event data in epidemiological studies is based on classification by variables of special medical interest. For births, the concern is with particular risk groups of newborn children, which may be defined by sex, birthweight, multiple births or place of residence, and age and parity of mothers. Classification of death involves even more varied subgrouping. It may reflect both past events in the life of the deceased and circumstances at the time of death. Besides the demographic variables of age, sex, place of residence, and time, there is, above all, classification by cause of death: the International Classification of Diseases (ICD) developed by the World Health Organization (WHO) is now accepted by most countries and is being revised for the ninth time. A more detailed description of this classification will follow.

Table 1 displays eight commonly used vital statistics for fifteen modern industrialized European countries. The table does not purport to compare conditions in these countries, but to illustrate the range of measurements in societies where there is a reasonable standard of living. The data are from 1971–1973, since these were the most recent obtainable from official reports at the time of writing.

Most of these measurements are of interest in demographic prediction and in health evaluation. The marriage rate is of historical interest but has limited value today. The lowest marriage rates are in Sweden and Denmark (4.8 and 6.2 respectively) but marriage rates currently bear little relation to measures of population growth or health, except perhaps for psychiatric disorders.

The fifteen countries are all characterized by low infant mortality rates, and by very low growth rates. Crude death rates are uncorrected for

Table 1. *Commonly used vital statistics for certain European Countries 1971–1973*
(*Source: Danmarks Statistik 1975*)

Country	Live birth rate	Repro- ductive rate i.e. fertility	Mar- riages	Crude death rate	Popula- tion over 65 years	Life ex- pectancy of males at birth	Infant mor- tality rate	Net growth rate
West Germany	10.2	750	6.7	11.8	134	67.4	23	−1.6
East Germany	10.6	766	7.8	13.7	158	68.5	16	−2.1
Austria	12.9	N.A.	7.6	12.3	145	66.6	24	0.6
Belgium	13.3	1075	7.7	12.1	135	67.8	17	1.2
Sweden	13.5	913	4.8	10.5	142	72.1	10	3.0
Switzerland	13.6	990	6.8	8.8	116	70.3	13	4.8
United Kingdom	13.9	981§	8.6	12.0	134	68.9§	17	1.9
Denmark	14.3	934	6.2	10.1	133	70.8	11	4.3
Finland	14.3	728	7.7	9.3	96	66.6	11	5.0
Netherlands	14.5	1061	8.8	8.2	104	70.8	12	6.3
Norway	15.5	1078	7.3	10.1	142	71.1	12	5.4
Italy	16.0	1157	7.7	9.9	107	67.9	26	6.1
France	16.4	1209	8.1	10.7	135	68.5	13	5.7
Iceland	21.5	1411	8.1	6.9	91	70.7	10	14.6
Ireland	22.5	N.A.	7.3	11.0	111	68.6	18	11.5
Median value	14.3	990	7.7	10.5	134	68.6	13	4.8

All rates are per 1000 population, except life expectancy which is in years
　§ England & Wales only　　N.A. = not available

population age distribution, so that the net growth rate can be directly calculated as the birth rate minus the crude death rate. Immigration data are not taken into account.

Crude death rates are naturally dependent on the age composition of the population. It is clear from Table 1 that the size of the population over 65 years is strongly correlated with crude death rates. Most of the countries in the table have high proportions of aged people. Age standardization of death rates is discussed later in this chapter.

USE OF BIRTH DATA

Data on the number of births can be used both as numerators and as denominators.

BIRTH RATES

As numerators, divided by various population counts, the total number of live births can be used to calculate crude birth rates (over total mid-year population), and fertility rates (over female population aged 15–44 years).

The use of these rates in studies of population dynamics is well known, text books of demography would give more details. More precisely defined are age-specific and parity-specific rates (often given in two-way tables). These rates are of use for developing an obstetric and paediatric health care programme, since they define maternal and infant risk groups. Complications at delivery tend to appear both in very young and in older mothers. Congenital anomalies are more common among infants born to older mothers and to multipara. In designing a community programme for prevention or *in utero* detection of such defects greatest cost-effectiveness is obtained by focusing attention in pregnancy on these high risk groups. This is particularly important when the anomalies are relatively rare and so cost of detection is high. There are of course numerous other examples of the use of specific birth rates.

PROPORTIONAL RATES

The relationship between live births and different variables may be examined and the proportion in each category expressed as a fraction of all live births. The sex of infants is a simple categorization of this type, for example, the proportion of boys may be 53 per cent. Often this particular distribution is described by the ratio of male to female births times 100 e.g. $(100 \times 53)/47 = 113$.

Prematurity rates are taken to be either the proportion of infants of given birthweight, or the proportion of infants that are deemed born 'before time'. The latter is less precise, and usually prematurity is defined by a birthweight of less than 2500 g. This is satisfactory for comparison of trends within the same population, but the cut-off point of 2500 g may not be appropriate to define prematurity in certain races and ethnic groups.

Illegitimacy rates give the proportion of live births that occur outside marriage. Nowadays this rate no longer bears such a strong moral allusion as it once did but illegitimacy remains as a measure of a group of infants who are at higher risk of death or under-development. Until this risk has declined markedly, it is a useful proxy variable, but it may disappear; in fact some countries do not permit reporting of 'illegitimate' births. Other variables such as maternal age may prove to be more precise measures of high risk but of a different type.

As demonstrated in Table 2, the risk of neonatal mortality is higher among children born outside marriage. However, the trend in Denmark over the last 15 years has been towards lower relative risks as more children are born to unmarried parents.

Table 2. *Neonatal mortality by marital status, Denmark 1961–1975 (Source: Danish National Health Service)*

Period	Married parents	Unmarried parents	Percentage of births to unmarried parents	Relative risk unmarried/married
1961–1965	14.0	25.4	8.8	1.81
1966–1970	11.3	18.7	10.9	1.65
1971–1975	8.4	10.1	16.7	1.20

DENOMINATOR RATES

The stillbirth rate is the number of stillbirths divided by all births, both live and dead delivered after the 28th week. It is not a good measure, because stillbirths are less completely reported than live births; because of greater precision in reporting live births, this count is used in all the following rates.

Infant and neonatal mortality are somewhat different in concept from other forms of age-specific mortality which is discussed later. While mortality is usually the number of deaths among persons with a particular characteristic divided by the number of persons supposed to be alive during the given period (usually a year), infant mortality is the number of live born children that die before their first birthday in a calendar year divided by the number of live births in the same year. Thus some individuals will appear in both the numerator and the denominator, but this has arisen for practical reasons. It is easier to obtain the number of live births than it is to get a census of live infants for a given year. Neonatal deaths, that is deaths within the first 28 days of life, are also divided by live births to form the neonatal death rate. In most modern communities the neonatal mortality rate is three-quarters of the infant mortality rate (Table 3).

The infant mortality rate has long been regarded as the most important and sensitive of all indices of community health, and it may well remain so for some time, since it is related to a number of social and economic variables as well as to the effectiveness of health care programmes.

Maternal mortality rates are deaths at puerperium divided by the total number of births (live and still) in the same time period. Again, the most precise number is used as the denominator, but since the numerator also contains deaths following abortion and stillbirths this must be taken into account.

Table 3. *Maternity and birth data, Denmark 1965–1974 (Source: Danish National Health Service)*

Year	Live births	Still-births	Legal abortions	Maternal deaths during		Infant neonatal mortality/1000	
				birth	abortion		
1965	85796	942	5188	8	4	18.7	14.4
1966	88332	875	5726	12	5	16.9	13.0
1967	81410	715	6324	6	2	15.8	12.3
1968	74543	636	5986	8	2	16.4	12.2
1969	71298	612	7295	9	3	15.8	12.3
1970	70802	604	9375	6	0	14.2	11.0
1971	75359	620	11157	4	0	13.5	10.7
1972	75505	577	12985	3	0	12.2	9.7
1973	71895	523	16536	2	0	11.5	8.7
1974	71327	441	24868	4	1	10.7	8.0

Table 3 gives the various rates over the last decade in Denmark. The abortion laws became more liberal in the late sixties and in 1973 'free' abortion, i.e. solely at the wish of the pregnant women, became legal. In 1974, about one-quarter of all pregnancies were terminated by legal abortion, 4.5 times more than 10 years earlier. Over the decade maternal deaths decreased, especially those ascribed to abortion. There was in fact only one such death from 1970 to 1974, as opposed to 16 abortion deaths in the previous five-year period.

This example illustrates the use of basic vital statistics in evaluation of a major socio-medical intervention.

In recent decades measurement of the abortion rate, has become more precise: in the past many natural and illegally induced abortions have not been recorded. Now, the legal abortion rate has become calculable by dividing reported operations by live births. This is obviously a ratio of the male/female type which will increase both as the number of abortions increases and as the number of live births decreases for that reason. The ratio might eventually become part of official vital statistics, and as such become an important life measurement and socio-medical index.

MORTALITY DATA

GENERAL MORTALITY

Crude mortality rate in a community is the total number of deaths in a year divided by the total population at mid-year. As this rate is approximately 10 per 1000 in most industrial nations, it has lost its significance as a health index. It reflects the causes of mortality at all ages, the composition of the population, and deaths from long-term chronic conditions which are the result of many factors acting over long periods. As an indicator of current health conditions, crude death rates are not sufficiently discriminating, and because most official reports are delayed for many years they only have retrospective interest. In the United States the Public Health Service collects current information on the progress of influenza epidemics by means of weekly reporting of all deaths from 118 cities. There are between 350 and 500 deaths from pneumonia in these cities every week, and major flu epidemics can cause significant variations from the expected weekly death rate, for which seasonal figures have been computed over 18 years.

Age-specific and sex-specific mortality rates are more suitable than crude death rates for the demonstration of health determinants. Age is probably the strongest covariant of mortality, and mortality data by age are among the most accurate and easily accessible vital statistics. And yet, age is only a proxy-variable that indicates areas of risk, but not causes of disease. In order to eliminate the association with age when comparing crude mortality of several populations, various statistical devices are used under the general term of 'age standardization'.

Direct standardization is traditionally the favoured method. Recognizing that various populations differ in their age composition, direct standardization uses a population with reasonable age-distribution and computes what the number of deaths in that population would be if the age-specific death rate of the studied populations was prevailing in that fictional population. Given that there are N_i individuals in the standard population at age i, and that deaths and persons at age i in the study population are d_i, and n_i respectively, then expected deaths in the standard population are computed as follows:

$$E(D) = \Sigma d_i \cdot N_i/n_i$$

By dividing the expected number of deaths with the total standard population one obtains a directly age-standardized mortality rate; this is

$$E(D)/\Sigma N_i$$

Application of this method to a number of population rates, for example the crude rates for a nation over a number of consecutive years, has enabled a set of standardized rates to be obtained where the influence

Table 4. *Deaths from cancer of the lung among cigarette smokers and non-cigarette smokers. Direct standardization to a normal population of males 45–79 years old* (*Source: American Cancer Society in* Smoking and Health)

Age at entry to study (i)	Non-cigarette smokers' deaths (d_i)	Population (n_i)	Cigarette smokers' deaths (d_i)	Population (n_i)	Standard population (N_i)
45–49	2	25 507	42	71 845	19 600
50–54	2	26 935	53	69 302	18 400
55–59	2	23 402	88	50 537	18 400
60–64	8	19 940	86	33 928	15 600
65–69	7	16 672	77	20 833	12 500
70–74	4	11 499	42	9 227	9 400
75–79	6	6 560	11	3 685	6 100
Total	31	130 515	399	260 057	100 000

Crude rate/ 100 000	23.8		153.4	Ratio: SM/N-S = 6.5
$\Sigma \dfrac{d_i N_i}{n_i}$	24.8		201.3	Ratio: SM/N-S = 8.1

of an age-shift in the population over time has been reasonably eliminated.

An example of direct age standardization is presented in Table 4. Between 1960 and 1962 the American Cancer Society interviewed about 400 000 adults to gather information about, among other things, smoking habits. Follow-up about 20 months later identified deaths from lung cancer. There were about twice as many deaths among cigarette smokers as among non-smokers or those who smoked cigars or a pipe. There were 399 deaths from lung cancer among smokers compared with 31 among non-smokers. The crude mortality rates are 153.4 and 23.8 respectively, giving a 6.5 times higher death rate for lung cancer in smokers than in non-smokers.

The age distributions of the two populations differed considerably— there were more at younger ages among the cigarette smokers implying that age standardization is relevant in this context. A standard population, based on the age distribution of European males aged 45–79, is used. Using the same method as before, we obtain E(D)/100 000 equal to 201.3 for smokers for 24.8 for non-smokers. The age-standardized mortality ratio smokers/non-smokers is now 201.3/24.8 = 8.1 which is markedly higher than the ratio using crude death rates.

It is always advisable to select a standard population that resembles the study population as closely as possible. A standard population in which the numbers in each age group, N_i, is the sum of the numbers of k study populations in that age group, so that $N_i = \Sigma_k n_{ik}$ for all age groups *i*, is preferable.

If for each age group, the sum of all deaths $D_i = \Sigma d_{ik}$ is found, it is possible to compute the ratio $100 \times E(D)/\Sigma D_i$, which is known as the Standard Rate Ratio (SRR).

The result of direct age standardization varies if a different standard population is used. If the sum of the two populations is used, as given in Table 5, the sums of expected deaths become 655.7 and 75.3, respectively, with standard mortality rates of 167.9 and 19.3. The ratio is now $167.9/19.3 = 8.7$. This is somewhat higher than the ratio of 8.1 that was obtained by comparison with a 'normal' population because the combined study population has a higher proportion of younger people than an average population. The SRR, with the sum of deaths being 430, would be 152.5 and 17.5.

Indirect standardization is a particularly useful method when mortality in two or more subgroups of a given population is to be compared. The total population has an age distribution with N_i members of the *i*th group. Also available are the figures for deaths in the total population for each age group, taken as D_i, each of which is the sum of deaths in the subgroups at that age. The indirect method calculates the number of deaths that would have occurred in a subpopulation if the age-specific mortalities of the total population were applied to the numbers in each age group of the subpopulation.

Expected deaths in the kth subpopulation is given by

$$E(d_k) = \Sigma n_{ik} \cdot D_i / N_i$$

This figure for expected deaths is compared to the observed numbers of deaths, $O(d_k) = \Sigma d_{ik}$. The result can be expressed by the ratio of observed over expected deaths, which multiplied by 100 is termed the Standard Mortality Ratio (SMR) $= 100 \cdot O(d_k)/E(d_k)$.

An illustration of indirect standardization is given in Table 5 using the data from Table 4. When mortality rates for each age of the total population are applied to the two populations expected deaths are 266.9 and 163.1, against observed deaths of 399 and 31. The SMRs are 149.5 and 19.0, and their ratio is now 7.9, which appears to be lower than those found by the two direct standardization methods.

The two methods of age standardization do not always give the same

Table 5. *Indirect standardization* (*Data from Table 4*)

Age	Non-cigarette smokers' deaths Observed (d_{i1})	Non-cigarette smokers' deaths Expected §	Cigarette smokers' deaths Observed (d_{i2})	Cigarette smokers' deaths Expected §	Total Deaths (D_i)	Total Population (P_i)
45–49	2	11.5	42	32.5	44	97 352
50–54	2	15.4	53	39.6	55	96 237
55–59	2	28.5	88	61.5	90	72 939
60–64	8	34.8	86	59.2	94	53 868
65–69	7	37.3	77	46.7	84	37 505
70–74	4	24.7	42	21.3	46	21 426
75–79	6	10.9	11	6.1	17	10 245
Observed deaths ($O(d_k)$)	31		399		430	
Expected deaths ($E(d_k)$)		163.1		266.9		430
SMR		19		149.5	Ratio:	7.9

§ Expected deaths = $D_i n_i / P_i$ (n_is are given in Table 4)

result, in that SMR and SRR may differ when calculated from the same set of mortality tables. However, there are three particular circumstances where SMR and SRR will give identical results:

1. When the study population has the same age-specific rates at all ages, that is $d_i/n_i = D_i/N_i$ for all *i*s. And hence SMR = SRR = 100.

2. When the age distribution of the study population is proportional to that of the standard population, that is n_i/N_i = constant for all age groups, SMR and SRR will both equal 100 times the ratio of the crude mortality rates for the two populations. It could be said that in this situation an age standardization is superfluous.

3. When every age-specific rate in the study population is proportional to that of the standard population by a constant factor, c, that is $d_i/n_i = c \cdot D_i/N_i$ for all age groups, both SMR and SRR will assume the value 100×c. This applies for condition 1, where c = 1.0.

If neither condition 2 nor condition 3 are fulfilled, direct and indirect standardization give different standard rates. This occurs, when the factor c is age dependent. There is no particular reason for saying that one method of age standardization is better than the other, both have their advantages and disadvantages. In case of disparity between the two standard rates one should assume that there is more information to be had from the data than a one-parameter statement such as SMR or SRR and more detailed analysis of the age/mortality relationship would be appropriate.

Comparison of mortality/age tables

Graphic presentation of mortality against age is an important means of hypothesizing about the relationship between the two variables. Logarithmic values for mortality rates are to be preferred, first because there is an enormous change in mortality by age, and secondly because two populations with different mortalities are best compared by inspection of log mortality data: differences will appear as the extent to which the two curves are paralleled.

It is well known that the curve for mortality over the different age groups is J-shaped with a minimum at about the age of 10 years, and that attempts to fit a simple mathematical formula for the whole curve must include a number of parameters. Over a rather extended—and particularly important—range from about 25 to 70 years of age the log mortality curve for general mortality and for a number of disease groups is almost a straight line. Over this range it is useful to express the difference in mortality experience in two populations by two parameters, the position and slope of the lines.

Life expectancy and age-survival curves

Life tables and life-expectancy parameters are based on the same concept as are age-standardized rates: several age-specific mortality rates of a population are combined by a prescribed method into one parameter, which purports to indicate the combined forces of mortality upon that population. (Details of the actuarial technique used will not be given here.) The restrictive assumptions underlying the life-expectancy indices are well known: one assumes that the age-specific mortality rates, that are prevailing in a given period will continue to exist for some years. So on that assumption it can be calculated how long a person aged x years still has left to live, or what the probability is that he will live to age y.

For populations with rapidly changing patterns of mortality, the absolute value of life-expectancy is of limited use. For the developed nations where life-expectancy from birth is about 70 years for males, life tables have a more realistic meaning. However useful they are for population predictions and assessment of insurance premium rates, life-expectancy as such is not really useful as a health index for epidemiological purposes. It is not sensitive enough for comparison of sections

Table 6. *Life expectancy table (abbreviated) for Denmark 1973–1974 (Source:* Statistisk Aarbog *1976)*

Age (x) (years)	Men		Women	
	Surviving at xth birthday	Life expectancy from age x (years)	Surviving at xth birthday	Life expectancy from age x (years)
0	100000	70.8	100000	76.6
1	98632	70.8	98990	76.4
5	98359	67.0	98794	72.5
10	98127	62.2	98659	67.6
15	97949	57.3	98536	62.7
20	97458	52.6	98338	57.8
25	96879	47.9	98126	52.9
30	96406	43.1	97911	48.0
35	95796	38.3	97543	43.2
40	94884	33.7	96942	38.5
45	93456	29.2	95894	33.8
50	91098	24.8	94196	29.4
55	87444	20.8	91870	25.1
60	81898	17.0	88465	20.9
65	73620	13.6	83624	17.0
70	61858	10.7	76591	13.3
75	47043	8.3	65978	10.0
80	31184	6.2	50351	7.3
85	16568	4.5	31671	5.2
90	6207	3.2	14250	3.6

of a modern population, and if differences are found, the components must be carefully scrutinized to identify the critical information.

Table 6 is abbreviated from a typical actuarial table which contains data for every year of life. The probability of living from birth to age x is given for each age by the survivors among 100000 births. In other words, for the given time and place, a man has a chance of 93456 in 100000 to live until his 45th birthday. A man aged 45 has a chance of 47043/93456 = 0.5 of surviving to age 75. These data make it possible to compare actual survival of a group of patients with their expected survival over a period of investigation. If, for example, out of 50 patients aged 55 at the start of treatment, 30 survived for 10 years, one would expect survival under 'natural conditions' to be 73620/87444 = 0.84, in other words 42 would survive from age 55 to 65.

In the epidemiology of chronic conditions the much-used *case fatality rate* (deaths among those with the disease divided by all those with the disease) has been partially replaced by the *survival curve*, which describes the probability of living x years after initial entry to a disease category. Essentially, this is a life table based on mortality by age after entry which is similar to mortality by age after birth: the difference lies in the way the mortality figures are obtained.

The survival curve enables the investigator to standardize the mortality among patients to some fixed point, for example, five-year survival, for which the method provides a standard error. In relation to construction of survival curves there has been much discussion about causes of death. It has been maintained that only deaths attributable to the disease should be included and, for example, deaths from other causes ('with the disease') should be excluded: in particular, it has been claimed that deaths due to treatment ('early operative mortality') ought to be excluded. The most reasonable procedure would be to include *all* deaths that occur in the study population: excluding treatment deaths would be equivalent to excluding infant mortality from a life expectancy calculation. The decision whether death occurs 'from' or 'with' the disease is fraught with subjective judgements.

The reasoning behind including all deaths is that chronically ill patients are subject both to the greater risk of mortality of the disease from which they suffer, and to the general risk of mortality which applies to everyone else. In order to separate the two types of risk one can calculate a survival curve for a population with the same age distribution as that of the patient population at the time of entry. The 'crude' five-year mortality rate can now be adjusted for age by dividing the observed survival rate of the patient population with the survival rate for the corresponding age distribution in the normal population. This method is of particular use in studies among older patients which run for a number of years.

In this method of age adjusting survival rates the empirical survival table technique is supported by the more theoretical national life tables which are part of official vital statistics. In selection of a standard life table population the same considerations apply as in age standardization of crude death rates. As for direct standardization, one can select the life table for the whole population of the same country for the period that falls in the middle of the period in which the study group was observed. Using the age distribution of the patients in the study group at time of entry, a survival curve for people of that age over the period of observation can be constructed. This is an easy task on a computer, but rather tedious manually.

If the period of observation extends over several decades, it may be necessary to use a combination of life tables for the whole period. This involves the use of the Lexis diagram technique. If, for example, a patient is a 40-year-old man when entered in the study in 1950, the life table for 40-year-old men for 1950 should be applied: if he is still alive in 1960, the life table for 50-year-olds for 1960 is used, and so on. By interpolation, one can refine the method by constructing life tables for every calendar year and then, so to speak, move the person to the next year's life table for each year he is alive.

Indirect life table standardization is used when survival curves for two or more study populations are compared. An extraneous life table is not necessary since the hypothesis to be tested is not as concerned with the force of mortality of the disease in question as with the differential risk between various forms of the disease (e.g. stages of cancer) or between the effect of various treatments on survival. Direct comparison of such individual study groups with the normal life table would only be necessary if the age distributions of the groups at entry varied greatly. With similar age groups at the start, as would apply in randomized controlled trials, the ratio of survival would be the chosen measurement. One can then either compare, say five-year survival data, or treat the mortalities by year after entry as sets of specific mortalities using exactly the same procedures as mentioned above for age-specific mortality comparison. The latter is particularly suitable for testing the hypothesis that the difference in effect of treatments or interventions is constant throughout follow-up.

DISEASE-SPECIFIC MORTALITY

The International Classification of Diseases (ICD) that has been developed over almost a century is an admirable testimony to international communication and cooperation. It is now possible for nearly every morbid condition known to modern medicine to be assigned a number between 000 and 999, and this number can be translated into a named disease in the language of any nation that has adopted the WHO/ICD coding. There are notable weaknesses: there is only limited systematic breakdown of disease types, if the first digit in the number is taken as a lead; causative agents (infections), pathology (malignancies), and anatomical sites are often interchanged; violent deaths are arranged in two different systems, the N-numbers (medical causes) and the E-numbers (social causes).

Yet, the system is vastly superior to a situation where every country uses different disease groupings, and where classifications change from year to year. Certainly, enough trouble arises each time the ICD system is revised, but it is possible to identify the changes from one published edition to the next. Difficulty arises not so much when a specified disease, for instance stroke, is allocated a new number but when an investigator is unaware that stroke has been moved from 'Diseases of the Central Nervous System' to 'Diseases of the Cardiovascular System'.

In general, the ICD system works reasonably well when interest is focused on a well-defined condition such as cancer of the lung, except that only national data is collected on such diseases, there are no breakdowns into smaller communities or social subgroups. The smaller the subgroup the less comprehensive is reporting by specific disease; for example, municipalities would not list 'Multiple Sclerosis', but only 'Diseases of the Nervous System', and probably not even list these by age or sex.

Hence, the usefulness of the ICD system is limited by the purpose and scope of the data to which it is applied. Consider, for example, that the purpose of a study is to identify the cause of excess deaths in a given population typified by a geographical or occupational setting. General mortality in that population may or may not show significant excess over that expected from national data, corrected for basic demographic variables. In either case, the investigator must set out to classify deaths by attributed cause. If there is no significant excess of total deaths, a smaller specific group of 'causes of death' may well reach the critical level of significance and thus indicate causative associations with the variables of the particular occupational or demographic setting.

If general mortality of the investigated group is significantly different from that expected, there is still reason to separate out the causes that are resulting in excess mortality in local groups. A hypothesis of abnormal exposure can be confirmed, if a mechanistic explanation can be found of why a certain pathological condition appears to be caused by a certain agent. Conversely, if no such reasonable causative mechanism can be found, the appearance of a cluster of specific diseases may enable revision of the hypothesis about the causative agent, and a new idea about causation could arise from knowledge of the aetiology of the disease for which the excess mortality has been demonstrated.

The many hundreds of items in the ICD may not always be useful in determining precise causes of death. The system, built on contemporary concepts of aetiology, needs constant revision and sometimes this does not cover new settings and causes of disease. For example, the causative association between lung cancer and cigarette smoking was strongly suggested in the early 1950s through retrospective case studies: subsequent prospective studies of populations defined by their smoking habits revealed other manifestations of cigarette smoking such as cancer of the bladder and coronary artery disease. In fact, the total impact of cigarette smoking can be measured in terms of excess general mortality, but the specific impact is best shown by aggregating a number of specific items in the ICD. Such *multiple manifestations* of a single cause dictates vigilant scrutiny of the disease categories that are most applicable to the problem at hand.

The contrasting principle of *multiple causes* of a defined disease has probably attained a more prominent position in the epidemiology of health care. It is recognized that a single causative mechanism rarely satisfies an aetiological hypothesis. The wealth of 'setting' variables of demographic and sociological derivation must be included in any explanatory concept. For an analysis of this kind the dependent variable—the disease—must be sharply defined, and for this purpose an itemized list of diseases using the ICD is particularly important.

PROPORTIONAL MORTALITY

There is still some fascination in studying causes of death simply by numbers of deaths in a population, listing them on a nominal scale and arranging them by the '10 most frequent' causes and 'the rest', and commenting on the predominance of a particular disease. This method precedes the era of age-specific and cause-specific mortality rates and in the past has led to some interesting conclusions: the pitfalls inherent in a comparison of populations on the basis of proportional mortalities are well-known. The most glaring bias is that a proportion of the cause of death in one population which seems to be in excess over another population may not be simply an excess of that cause, it may result from under-representation of another cause. If for example, in one population, cancer appears to be more common, but at the same time deaths from heart disease are less common than in another population, which is the most important finding—excess of cancer or deficit of heart disease? Mortality rates adjusted appropriately to age, sex and other variables, would be essential to expand the study to answer the question satisfactorily.

On the other hand, proportional distribution of causes of death does illustrate the important health problems in a population.

SUGGESTED TEXTS FOR BACKGROUND READING

Boyne, J. D. (1969) *Principles of Demography*. New York: John Wiley

Danish National Health Service (1976 and other years) *Causes of Death in Denmark*. Copenhagen

Ipsen, J. & Feigl, P. (1970) Chapters 11–14. In Bancroft's *Introduction to Biostatistics*. New York: Harper & Row

Mausner, J. S. & Bahn, A. K. (1974) Chapters 7–10. In *Epidemiology. An Introductory Text*. Philadelphia: Saunders

Smoking and Health (1964) Report of the Advisory Committee to the Surgeon General of the Public Health Services, United States Department of Health, Education and Welfare. USPHS Publication number 1103. Washington D.C., US Government Printing Office

Statistisk Aarbog. (1976 and other years) Danmarks Statistik, Copenhagen

CHAPTER 4

Health Information Systems

Maarten Hartgerink

The concept of a health information system incorporates a continuous flow of specified information and the possibility of integrated presentation of facts from different sources. There may be epidemiological reasons for setting up a health information system as well as a general medical purpose related to a disease and treatment of patients. However, the primary purpose, together with a medical purpose, may well be the need for operational information about health care delivery.

Different sources and types of information can be distinguished and there is a close relationship between the type of information collected and the use to which it will be put. Information requirements vary with the organizational level of the health service: the higher levels usually require less detail than the levels at which health care is delivered. Some examples of health information systems are given.

Certain conditions have to be fulfilled for any system to be reliable and effective and some emphasis is placed on the importance of protection of privacy both for patients and doctors. Those setting up health information systems have certain responsibilities in this respect.

DEFINITION

The meaning of the term 'health information system' is better given by common understanding than by precise definition. For the word 'system' alone most definitions given are similar to 'any whole from the standpoint of the methodic connection and arrangement of its constituent members'. Even so the word is sometimes given very different meanings depending on whether the natural coherence of the components is stressed or the emphasis is placed on the operational principle for the specific purpose.

For the purpose of this book an attempt by the World Health Organization (WHO) to define a health information system seems adequate: 'A mechanism for the collection, processing, analysis and transmission of information required for organizing and operating health services, and also for research and training' (WHO 1973). But not every means of systematic collection of medical data should be called a health information system; if this were so, the medical record for every patient would come under this heading. The term 'health information system' should be reserved for data collection that serves a more general purpose than direct medical treatment. As a rule such a system will combine information from different sources; for example, disease characteristics, indications on the course of treatment and organizational aspects of patient handling (Figure 1, p. 53). Thus the system provides a powerful epidemiological tool: it can form the base for good general statistics and an adequate source of management information.

GOALS

In the practice of medicine recollection of previous experience and collection of information has always existed: certainly in the 19th century a lot of information from different sources in medical and social fields was systematically brought together to the advantage of decision making in public health and the treatment of individual patients. But both the expansion of medicine as a science and the increasing complexity of the organization of health care delivery have resulted in the task of mastering the increasing flow of information by carefully selecting and integrating the relevant facts. 'Information is the essential ingredient in decision making. The need for improved information systems in recent years has been made critical by the steady growth in size and complexity of organizations and data' (Rosove 1967).

One of the goals for a health information system is to provide a doctor with the type of information that will help him take the best possible decision about any single patient under his care. The other goal lies in the fact that effective functioning of health administration, of planning and of control demands readily available information and that this information is indispensable for adequate policy making. The delivery, evaluation and control of the health care system is not possible without the aid of reliable information about the functioning of the system. Equally, the collection, processing and analysis of data becomes imperative for providing guidelines for planning, for rules and regulations relevant in effective and comprehensive operation of the health care system and for norms governing the quality of health services. Epidemiology, whether it is briefly defined as the study of the distribution and determinants of disease in man (MacMahon and Pugh 1970; Kark 1974), or more broadly defined to include the determinants of the course of diseases (Hartgerink 1972b), is dependent on the proper availability of information. Hence the interest of epidemiologists in health information systems: in fact their use in epidemiology may well be one of the major scientific goals for any system.

These are in general terms the goals for health information systems but it should be stressed that the goals to be achieved by setting up such a system must be specified clearly and in detail for each case before any development takes place. The design of a system with the primary objective of providing doctors with the type of information required for day-to-day practice would differ greatly from the design of one with the objective of providing managers, administrators and planners with information relevant to them. Under certain conditions the requirements of both can be brought together in one system: but generally it is difficult to combine the details of medical observations and treatment necessary for in-depth pathological studies with wider overall information usually required by administrators and planners. In reality a health information system, whether automated or not, should only be set up after careful consideration of its goals and the demands of its users (Brauers 1976; Atsumi and Kaihara 1975).

SOURCES

The sources which can provide an input into a health information system appear to be manifold. From the epidemiological point of view birth certificates, medical records of sickness episodes, death certificates, notification of disease and special disease registers, insurance registers and population registers can all be considered as possible sources of information which can be transferred to a health information system. But also facts from morbidity surveys and special investigations or even the results of screening in sections of the population can provide material for a more integrated health information system. Health administrators will often be interested in, say, general operational information from health services and their financial implications.

This diversity of sources and the need for generally available methods of control, surveillance and investigation of data input do pose organizational problems when considering the scope and structure of a health information system. Most of the strictly *medical* information can only be obtained from places where primary health care is delivered or from hospitals. If the system is to cover an area or even a larger region it is a substantial task to bring all the sources together in a cooperative effort to ensure that the system works. An example of how this can be considered as an array of several dozen information sources linked to a 'master patient register' is described and illustrated by Bodenham and Wellman (1972). But such an elaborate system has not as yet been undertaken and it is not known if such a complex design on that scale would work in practice. The basic questions to answer are what type of information and how much of it should be integrated into the system, and what is its intended use. A carefully considered selection of contents and sources is essential for any satisfactory system.

As will be seen later in this chapter it is important to decide if the facts from some sources should be handled as a partly autonomous subsystem or even perhaps pooled entirely separately in such a way that they can still be called on occasionally or at defined intervals to be linked with the main system. In nearly every country this would apply to data from legally prescribed procedures, such as notification of births and deaths and the general population register. Also, if you can rely on the completeness and the accuracy of the sources, it is unnecessary for the central part of the system to contain the same detail as is contained in the contributing sources.

TYPES OF INFORMATION

There are two main categories of information gathered on health care: one is the facts directly related to the condition of the individual patient and the other comprises data from the organization of health care delivery. It should be noted that epidemiology and operational research (or management control) must draw information from both categories. Some people consider that there is a third category of information, which is the services rendered directly to the patient: these have a direct medical significance but at the same time they can be regarded as an organizational item. Figure 1 shows how these categories of information can be seen as both separate and interrelated: the two main lines can lead to reporting and archiving for each of them. It will often prove useful to report on the basis of facts from both streams of information and for planning purposes mixed reporting is essential. The facts directly related to the conditions of the individual patient together with his identifying characteristics are usually called the medical record. There is substantial

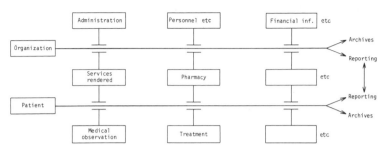

Figure 1. Main streams in a health information system

literature on the topic of the medical record, most of which is about hospital in-patient records. This results from many years of ongoing discussion about the medical record and shows how difficult it is to decide what should be the formalized content of a medical record. Most doctors and certainly all specialists make notes about the patient's history and the findings during observation and examination and about the outcome of treatment. But how much of this should be kept and fed into a central health information system? There is still no agreement on the ideal medical record for general use (Central Health Service Council 1965; Hartgerink 1975).

From a purely medical point of view this uncertainty about the medical record as part of the health information system is not surprising. There is considerable variation in the way doctors in different specialties describe the development of a disease. It would be unreasonable to expect, say, a dermatologist to use the same phrases for his findings in a patient as a physician or a neurologist. One way out of this dilemma is to choose a restricted summary of the medical data. Sometimes this is described as the 'minimum basic data set' (US National Committee on Vital and Health Statistics 1972; De Heaulme 1973). With the greatest emphasis placed on medical findings many hospitals already use a standardized 'hospital discharge summary' as an important part of the input to their hospital information system (Wagner, Immick and Kohler 1968; Griesser 1973; Van Egmond 1974; Wagner 1976); see also Table 1.

Information collection from primary health care engenders quite different problems when it is intended for use in a health information system. Certain preventive activities in primary health care such as vaccinations given, specific diagnostic tests performed or diagnoses which can be considered as hard fact are all valuable contributions to epidemiology; but much of the work and observation which takes place in primary

Table 1. *Uses made of the hospital discharge summary forms*

Uses	No. of answers	%
1 Hospital activity statistics	77	85
2 Hospital operation and management studies	44	48
3 Hospital planning	38	42
4 Administrative purpose	47	52
5 Epidemiological research	55	60
6 Patient scheduling	11	12
7 Forwarding information to physician	32	35
8 Entering information in data bank	45	49
9 Other	17	19
Total number of answers	366	
Number of respondents	91	100.0

medical care is not easily defined in precise diagnostic terms or in specific treatment activities. In the contact between patient and general practitioner or public health nurse many general impressions and preliminary findings precede an eventual diagnosis and quite often no diagnosis at all is reached. It is certainly difficult to feed formalized reports of such medical transaction into an information system. Several attempts have been made to do so (Bradshaw-Smith 1976; Van der Kooy 1975) but in terms of a more integrated health information system they have not been very successful. On the other hand it is often claimed that pooling of information from primary medical care may lead to a better understanding of early symptoms and development of disease. However, for this purpose the best approach would be to deal with this relatively 'soft' information in a separate information system.

THE USE OF HEALTH INFORMATION SYSTEMS

There are three main domains where health information systems have been successfully developed: epidemiology, management and planning. Later chapters in this book deal extensively with epidemiology and the material which forms the basis of this discipline and many of the facts the epidemiologist draws upon can, of course, be collected, stored and compiled in health information systems. There are good examples of special systems created for epidemiological purposes: disease registers, health surveys, information pooling in special investigations, etc. These special systems are not themselves regarded as health information systems, but they can be part of a more complex system of recording the findings in a population. Perhaps it is appropriate to distinguish between general or integrated health information systems and these more specific systems.

Accurate recording of sickness episodes and storage of such records is of value for future treatment of the individual patients: in this way a health information system is of use to the individual doctor.

To provide support for management and planning activities is often the goal when a health information system is established. The underlying idea is that a mixture of information from the organization of the services and from medical reports on patients can provide a better understanding of real needs, the usage and efficiency of the health care provisions.

A recent survey by WHO in the European Region has shown how information from hospital discharge summaries has actually been used (Wagner 1976).

LEVELS OF USE

The various uses of health information systems that have been described indicate that use will vary at different levels of the organization of the health services. All information is of course generated at the level of actual health care delivery, but some of it is only meaningful at certain levels of administration, control and planning. On the other hand much of what is relevant at the lowest executive level will only partly serve a purpose at the coordinating level and for the policy making levels still further selection will be required. As much consideration must be given to item selection for use at higher levels of the system as is given to items for primary input (De Paula 1966; Hartgerink 1975).

It might also be envisaged that some items of information from the primary input will only be collected in a specific 'line' for a particular purpose. This 'splitting of the system' about the level of primary input is of particular interest to health economists (Lièss 1976) and it can also be used by epidemiologists and for other specific purposes. Figure 2 illustrates a model of such a system.

EXAMPLES OF HEALTH INFORMATION SYSTEMS

In many countries the concept of a health information system is, at least partially, understood. Particularly in the hospital field a number of advanced developments have been shown to work, and there have also been developments in the sphere of general practice. These developments have led several computer companies to introduce small computer sys-

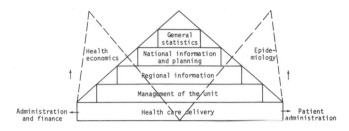

Figure 2. A model for the use of health information on different levels
and for different purposes

tems with programs which enable automation of a number of chosen
functions. One can consider health information systems without implying
the need for electronic data processing but full development of large
comprehensive information systems is becoming ever more dependent
on computers.

For illustrative purposes there follow some examples of information
systems that have been put into practice. It is important to realize that
the approach may be 'downwards' from centrally pooled information to
the level of primary data collection, or it can be 'upwards', from the health
care delivery level to the central or even national users of the information.
If we illustrate what can be achieved at a medical practice level the links
with the general management and planning level should be borne in mind.
Technically there are two alternative methods of providing this linkage:
the peripheral health care delivery point may only be responsible for input
of information to the system, if automated techniques are used this will
be by way of a terminal; or the peripheral unit will have its own information processing facilities, in computer system terminology this is called
distributed processing. Again, it is worth noting that automation is not
essential, handwritten documents may serve the purpose just as well.

A GENERAL PRACTITIONER UNIT
In group practices or community health centres it may be useful to store
and distribute information from the different activities in and around the
health centre. At the large health centre run by Philips Industries at
Eindhoven (Netherlands) an information system (code-name MICOS) has
been developed and put into practice (Figure 3). It is easy to understand
how this self-contained system could be partially linked to regional or
national information systems. This system has proved to be rather
expensive but it illustrates what can be achieved to serve both doctors

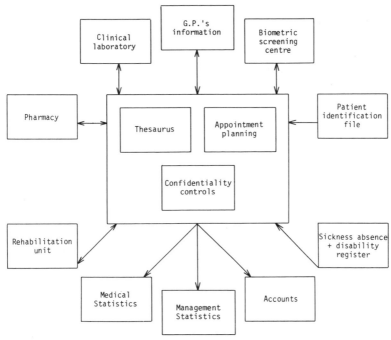

Figure 3. System with subsystems in a large general practitioner's unit at an industrial plant (Source: MICOS by Corporate ISA-Philips, Eindhoven)

in practice and the organizations responsible for operational control, planning and epidemiological surveillance. However, a major problem remains: in general practice it is difficult to achieve the level of formality of information items essential for central pooling of information on a national scale.

HOSPITAL INFORMATION
Since the early sixties a number of hospital information systems have been developed which perform a variety of functions. They all cling to the same basic principle which is that patient registration is the axis to which treatment and service information are linked. The effectiveness of this principle is illustrated in the use that is made of the system by the various wards and departments which mostly require medical information about the individual patient, and by the administrative information that becomes available to the hospital management. Such integrated hospital

information systems do require quite complex computer systems which are expensive to develop but cheap to run when installation is complete. Their advantages and disadvantages both in functional value to the hospital and from an economic viewpoint are difficult to calculate.

An integrated hospital information system can serve as a sound data collection system for use at a patient level but for the general purposes of management, planning and epidemiology a much more modest way of collecting information from the hospital is sufficient. The English National Hospital Survey and the Dutch Medical Registration Centre for hospitals (SMR) are examples of a much more restricted but nevertheless effective way of using information from hospitals for general purposes.

REGIONAL OR NATIONAL HEALTH INFORMATION SYSTEMS

In most developed countries a wide variety of information 'packages' are available to national authorities. This collection of information packages is not often regarded as a health information system because traditionally the different types of information have been collected in different organizational structures. Development into health information systems is well under way in several European countries: the continuous flow of specified information from the health care delivery and its organization is gradually brought together under one organizational set-up and can be integrated with information from vital statistics, social welfare and population census. This development has been described in the Bodenham and Wellman report (1972). A good example is to be found in Scotland, which is described as follows in a WHO report:

'The present health information system in Scotland has slowly evolved from a situation where vital statistics and limited health services data were mainly required for central government purposes and as a matter of historical record towards a system when information for monitoring, evaluation, planning and management of health services is more readily available in proper form. The Information Services Division of the Common Services Agency has the task of providing a service for production of information used in the planning, management and administration of the health service.' (WHO 1977).

Although in this description of the systematic approach to health information in Scotland there is no mention of epidemiological point of view, one may hope and expect that this approach would be of use to descriptive epidemiology. In any case it should lead to a system as depicted in the diagram in Figure 2.

Armitage (1977) has collected together papers by a variety of authors who describe the various health surveys and resulting information systems in all the EEC countries and the US. This provides a useful text for comparing and contrasting systems that have been used in the past or are in general use at the moment.

CONTINUOUS AND DISCONTINUOUS INFORMATION

Perhaps the computer era has led to overemphasis of the use of continuous streams of information. But in certain circumstances there are a number of advantages inherent in immediate input of facts and observations to a health information system: direct input into a computer terminal may eliminate the need for intermediate information carriers in the form of coded or uncoded written statements; and a further advantage is that a statement of the information in the system is readily available. Normally however there is little need for an immediate input process and in most cases a reasonable delay is acceptable which then allows batch-processing to take place. At the health care delivery level there is often a need for readily available information about individual patients from the information system and this has led to the concept of medical data banks. Basically these are stores of predominantly medical information about individual patients which can be readily consulted at any time. However, at other levels of administration or planning this instant availability of information is rarely necessary.

Whenever a health information system is being set up a decision must be made about input and availability of information. The following scheme illustrates the main possibilities:

continuous ⎫   ⎧ direct on request
discontinuous ⎬ input—availability ⎨ periodical
periodical ⎭   ⎩ on request with a delay

However, there is also a more fundamental issue affecting the choice between continuous and discontinuous input in a health information system. Often facts collated from a continuous flow of information are presented in such a form so as to relate them to the situation on a given date. For example, calculation of the incidence of a disease over a period relates the number of cases of the disease to the total population: in practice epidemiologists will accept a population figure for a certain date if it can be assumed that over the period that the cases of disease were notified no significant change in the population occurred. However, this assumption is not always justified: especially when factors related to organization of the health service are involved it is essential to verify if the number or the value of such factors (e.g. number of personnel or hospital beds available) have remained relatively stable for the period during which the continuous count of study items took place.

PREREQUISITE CONDITIONS

An information system brings together a great many facts of different type and origin. It is essential that all personnel contributing to the system use exactly the same words and have the same understanding of their meaning. Uniformity of definition is vital for a good information system. If figure values are used there must be absolute uniformity in the underlying measurement but unfortunately this principle is often disregarded. For instance, one hospital may count the number of days for treatment of a patient including the first and the last day, whereas another hospital may subtract the day of discharge or admission and so will count one day less: in this way the total count of bed-usage and mean values of duration of stay in hospital will differ considerably.

Uniformity of definitions and of measurement are the corner-stones of any information system and of accurate statistics. Several techniques have been introduced to ensure these conditions are fulfilled. Agreement on classifications for diagnoses and for medical procedures has been furthered by WHO and this work has laid the basis for some fairly reliable international health statistics. But there are still several subjects, particularly in relation to health service organization, that cannot yet be compared on an international basis. The use of coding systems is yet another way to make information homologous and to formalize it and they are of particular value in automated data processing: however, there is very little uniformity among coding systems. When setting up a health information system it is essential that the coding system to be used is selected beforehand.

Much of the work of an epidemiologist is in safeguarding the quality of the primary data. When data are brought into a health information system it is essential that classifications, codes and handling procedures used will ensure that the quality of the information meets the highest possible standards of uniformity and reliability.

INTEGRATION OF FACTS FROM DIFFERENT SOURCES

It is remarkable that in the field of health care in the last 20 years so much attention has been given to record linkage as a new technique. In essence it is only a better and more formal method of collating various aspects of the life history of a patient. As such it is exactly the same as 'taking the patient's history' which has been practised in medicine ever since Hippocrates' time. In medical literature the term 'record linkage' was used for the first time by Dunn in 1946 who was then head of the National Office of Vital Statistics in the USA. He proposed that far more use could be made of statistics of birth and death if facts from different sources could be linked: 'It would greatly enhance the significance of such statistics if they could be linked to other facts about the same individuals, such as, what sort of jobs do they hold, how many children do they have, what sort of illness did they suffer from, what kind of social environment do they live in?' (Dunn 1946). In Europe several others, and especially Acheson, have contributed to the acceptance of this viewpoint in health care and to the necessary techniques. Acheson defined medical record linkage as '. . . the process of bringing together selected data of biological interest for a population commencing with the conception and ending in death, into a series of personal cumulative files, the files being so organized that they can also be assembled in family groups' (Acheson 1967). Record linkage has opened up several possible perspectives in relation to solution of particular problems. One particular example is the study of the development of disease in individuals, taking account of family relationships and associations between diseases and social factors (Hartgerink 1972a).

In discussing health information systems we accept that a number of different sources will contribute to the system (see page 51). If the individual patient remains recognizable by name or code when information is brought together from different sources record linkage does, in fact, take place.

When no proper integration of personal files is contemplated within the health information system data will be combined from different sources for the compilation of statistics. If these sources are not already independently organized a good solution is to handle a specific source as a subsystem with both an independent aim and a contributory function in the main system (Härö 1976).

PRIVACY AND RESPONSIBILITY

The development of integrated health information systems has created the problem of privacy for the individual—what and how much do we allow other people and public administration to know about us?

In complex modern society for purposes of the administration of taxes, social assistance, health care, etc. the individual is unable to avoid revealing certain conditions of his personal life and status. He has to accept that to some extent decisions are taken on the basis of his personal information. This need for information should not encroach on the rights and independence of the individual and it may even be used to his advantage as an instrument of legal security and equality before the law. Thus the individual is not really in a position to claim an absolute right to his privacy.

In relation to medical care every patient has in the past accepted that his doctor keeps a record about his health. But since the medical profession and the health administration increasingly claim better medical care can be delivered if more is known about treatment and previous treatments of a patient, many individuals have started to ask how much private information should be revealed to members of medical professions and to administrators. The concepts of the progress of socio-medical care and of the science of medicine are considered to be too vague to be valid without restrictions on pooling identifiable personal medical information in a health information system. The problem of confidentiality of personal data collected by a number of agencies is now a matter of great concern.

It is worth noting that the introduction of computers for information systems has influenced the situation regarding privacy in two ways. On one hand the handwritten medical record can be read more easily, and thus misused by unqualified people, than a computer memory but, on the other hand, a computer-based system concentrates so much personal information that many people's interests may be affected by a security breakdown. In addition a computer-based system may well combine information from different sources making possible encroaches on privacy even more obvious.

Several techniques can be used to safeguard privacy in health information systems. The main ones are:

1. Omitting the name of the patient and of the unit where the health care was given. These can be replaced by identification numbers which are only known outside the system itself. There are several different ways

Information levels

Users	Medical record	Summary record	Anonymus record	Statistical presentation
Patient	✕	Through own doctor	✕	✕
Doctor in charge	Unrestricted	ibid.	ibid.	ibid.
Department of treatment	✕	Unrestricted	ibid.	ibid.
Research personnel	Without patient identity	ibid.	ibid.	ibid.
National Health Authorities	✕	✕	Unrestricted	ibid
Other institutes	Under special arrangement	Under special arrangement	Unrestricted	ibid.

Figure 4. Example of a confidentiality matrix for a health information system

of creating personal numbers for use instead of names: they may be completely unique or comprise of a combination of personal characteristics like age, sex and date of birth. The degree of 'selectivity' of the created number must be calculated in order to avoid misrouting of information about an individual. Sometimes a combination of the two methods of deciding on a number is preferable. Whenever numbers instead of names are used it must be remembered that few patients will know their personal 'health care number': this means they will have to carry their number with them on a written document which introduces a security risk.

2. An alternative safeguard against abuse of personal records is in the use of secret call-numbers for qualified users in their communications with the information system. In practice these secret call-numbers soon become known to people other than the qualified user (be it only the secretary).

3. A further safeguard, but really more a matter of principle, is that different types of personal record should not be brought together in one information system, for example judicial records and medical records should not be combined. In several countries legislation prohibits such combinations and supervisory boards have been set up to enforce and control the measures to safeguard the privacy of the individual.

But whatever official rulings and legally implemented safeguards there are it is of great importance that at the level of the primary data collection all those involved in health care delivery and the reporting of it should adhere to a formal system in this respect. To maintain discipline in security matters it might be useful to draft a 'confidentiality matrix', which would give precise instructions about which information may be made available to whom. It is essential that the matrix is appropriate to the situation in the unit for which it is intended. An arbitrary example is illustrated in Figure 4.

A health information system is a powerful tool in the advancement of medical knowledge, in health surveillance and the management of health services. However, as the above text has described, implementation of such systems increases the responsibility of the medical profession for the welfare and privacy of the individual patient.

REFERENCES

Acheson, E. D. (1967) *Medical Record Linkage*. London: Oxford University Press

Armitage, P. (ed.) (1977) *National Health Survey Systems in the European Economic Community. Proceedings of a conference held in Brussels, 6–8 October 1975*. Luxembourg: Commission of the European Communities

Atsumi, K. & Kaihara, S. (1975) Planning a national medical information system. In *Systems Aspects of Health Planning*. Bailey, N. T. J. & Thompson, M. (editors). Amsterdam: North-Holland Publishing Company

Bodenham, K. & Wellman, F. (1972) *Foundations for Health Service Management*. London: Oxford University Press

Bradshaw-Smith, J. H. (1976) A computer record-keeping system for general practice. *British medical Journal, 1*, 1395

Brauers, K. M. (1976) *Systems Analysis, Planning and Decision Models*. Amsterdam: Elsevier

Central Health Service Council. (1965) *The Standardization of Hospital Medical Records*. London: Central Health Service Council

De Heaulme, M. (1973) Archivage et interrogation de dossiers évolutifs. *Revue Information Médicale, 4*, 201

De Paula, W. (1966) In: Report of the British Joint Computer Conference, Eastbourne 1966. In *The Place of the Computer in the Delivery of Health Care*. (Cited by Barber, B.) Univac.

Dunn, H. L. (1946) Record linkage. *American Journal of Public Health, 36*, 1412

Griesser, G. (1973) Ansätze zu einem Gesundheits Informations-system

in Schleswig-Holstein. In *Computer, Aufgaben im Gesundheits-wesen.* p. 88. Hollberg, N. (ed). Berlin: Springer
Härö, A. S. (1976) Strategies for the development of health related statistics. In *Cross-national Sociomedical Research, Concepts, Methods, Practice.* Pflanz, M. & Schach, E. (eds). Stuttgart: Thieme
Hartgerink, M. J. (1972a) Record linkage, verbinding van intermitterende ziektegeschiedenissen. In *Computer en Medische Zorg*, p. 118. Leiden: Stafleu
Hartgerink, M. J. (1972b) Epidemiologisch onderzoek van bevolkings-groepen. *Tijdschrift voor sociale Geneeskunde, 50*, 935
Hartgerink, M. J. (1975) Traitement automatique des données cliniques. *Nouvelles Techniques, 4*, 109
Kark, S. L. (1974) *Epidemiology and Community Medicine.* New York: Appleton-Century-Crofts
Liëss, M. (1976) *Economical Aspects of Central Record Systems.* What the economist can expect from a centralized hospital data system. Edinburgh: Workshop on hospital statistics of the European Economic Communities
MacMahon, B. & Pugh, Th. F. (1970) *Epidemiology, Principles and Methods.* Boston: Little Brown
Rosove, P. E. (1967) *Developing Computer-based Information Systems.* New York: Wiley
U.S. National Committee on Vital and Health Statistics (1972) Uniform hospital abstract, minimum basic data set. Rockville, Md. *Vital and Health Statistics*, Series 4, number 14
Van der Kooy, S. (1975) Registratie van medische gegevens door de huisarts. *Huisarts en Wetenschap, 18*, 261
Van Egmond, J. & Wieme, R. J. (1974) Belgian inter-university project on computerization of the medical record. *Medinfo*, p. 45
Wagner, G., Immick, M. & Köhler, C. (1968) Der Krankenblattkopf der Heidelberger Kliniken. *Methods of Information in Medicine, 7*, 17
Wagner, G. (1976) *Uses of the Hospital Discharge Summary Forms in the European Region.* Copenhagen: World Health Organization
WHO (1973) *Health information systems. Report on a conference.* Copenhagen: World Health Organization
WHO (1977) *Information systems in the health services.* Copenhagen: World Health Organization

SUGGESTED TEXTS FOR BACKGROUND READING

Hogerzeil, H. H. W., Nielen, G. C., Tuinstra, C., Hempenius, K., Scholtis, J. H., Beukers, H. R., Meijler, F. L., Strackee, J., Hugenholtz, P. G., Miller, A. C., De Groote, V. A., Fokkens, O., Hartgerink, M. J., De Groot, M. J. W. & Vinken, P. J. (1972) *Computer en medische zorg.* Leiden: Stafleu Nederlanse bibliotheek de geneeskunde

Holland, W. W. (1970) *Data handling in epidemiology*. London: Oxford
  University Press
Schneider, B. & Schönenberger, R. (1976) *Datenverarbeitung im Gesund-
  heitswesen. Erreichtes und Geplantes*. Berlin: Springer
Selbmann, H. K., Überla, K. & Greiller, R. (1976) *Alternativen mediz-
  inischer Datenverarbeitung. Fachtagung, München-Grosshadern, 19
  February 1976*. Berlin: Springer

CASE-CONTROL STUDIES

CHAPTER 5

Case-Control Studies

Claude Rumeau-Rouquette

This classical epidemiological technique used to test causal hypotheses compares a group suffering from a particular condition with a control group, both groups being alike in a number of respects.

A number of problems arise in such studies. If a study takes place in a hospital both groups of patients (cases and controls) should be comparable in terms of their admission rate to hospital; to ensure this it may be necessary to use several control groups: studies which take place in the general population are thus preferable. When interview techniques are used errors between the two groups will vary. In statistical analysis only the relative risk from an aetiological factor can be calculated rather than the actual risk. The reasonable cost of these studies often mean they are the method of choice but controls are often less adequate than in prospective studies.

INTRODUCTION

Retrospective studies are among the classical epidemiological methods. They include prevalence surveys, performed on the total population or a representative sample (Butler and Alberman 1969; Rumeau-Rouquette et al 1976), and case-control studies. In this book prevalence studies are considered in Section 4, so only case-control studies are described here: their applications to the aetiology of disease and to health care are described.

AIMS OF CASE-CONTROL STUDIES

Research into causation of disease is one of the primary aims of case-control studies. In the field of infectious disease they have enabled sources of infection to be detected quickly and the vectors identified. They have also contributed to the explanation of certain rare and accidental phenomena such as the increase in cases of phocomelia related to the administration of thalidomide in the first trimester of pregnancy.

With regard to more common non-infectious diseases, there has been some success in research into the causes of cancer and this has often involved epidemiologists. It has been possible to isolate aetiological factors such as tobacco by questioning various types of cancer patient and comparing them with controls.

However, research into causation has encountered many obstacles which arise because observation studies are unable to provide a definite conclusion about causation and because of the limitation of retrospective studies which are plagued by considerable mistakes and omissions on questionnaires.

In view of the first problem, aetiological research has turned to the identification of risk factors in order to detect high risk populations and so introduce appropriate preventive measures. Case-control surveys have contributed to the isolation of risk factors and to the calculation of relative risk in population groups.

Difficulties are also encountered in investigation of risk factors. There are restrictions in applying the notion of risk to health improvement programmes and thus investigation of risk factors may prove useless and even dangerous if preventive methods are unknown and even if they are known their introduction may be difficult because of opposition from the medical profession and the public (Rumeau-Rouquette et al 1976).

In recent years a third aspect of case-control studies has been in the planning and evaluation of health programmes; thus case-control studies may facilitate the reorganization or development of preventive and treatment services rather than relying on direct reporting by these services. This aspect will be considered in the next chapter.

TARGET POPULATION FOR SURVEY AND SAMPLING METHODS

CHOICE OF THE TARGET POPULATION (Rumeau-Rouquette and Schwartz 1970)

(a) *Target population defined on an administrative basis, independent of the disease*

Examples are studies carried out in a whole country, region or town. These studies depend on the systematic registration of new cases (incidence) or existing cases (prevalence) of disease or deaths. In Stewart's survey (1958) of the aetiology of leukaemia each child who died of the disease was matched with a child of the same age and sex and born in the same district. When registration does not exist it is necessary to draw up lists of patients in the study before carrying out investigations. This is somewhat cumbersome although certain circumstances will make it simpler: in many countries these surveys are relatively easy at the time of birth, when the mother is admitted to hospital, or surveys can be carried out during school years or at the time of army call-up.

(b) *Target population defined by disease category*

These surveys are carried out in hospitals where patients are compared with controls admitted to hospital for other reasons. These studies, despite being easy to conduct, suffer from substantial error (Berkson 1946). In a survey conducted by the author, women with cervical cancer were compared with matched controls admitted to the same hospital for benign diseases. Statistical analysis showed that the cancer patients were of higher social class and had fewer children than the controls. These results, which contrasted directly with those of other surveys, were obtained because the controls were recruited from the lowest social classes, whereas the cancer patients were fairly representative of all cases of cervical cancer in the population. So in this example, aetiological factors were also factors affecting hospital admission.

In addition since the controls used are patients themselves, they could be suffering from disease connected with the aetiological factors being studied. For example the comparison of cancer patients with controls suffering from other conditions in respect of their alcohol consumption tends to reduce the apparent differences since alcohol is the cause of a number of diseases and aggravates many others (Tuyns, Jensen and Pequignot 1977).

Several solutions have been put forward to avoid these errors which seriously affect the interpretation of results. The first is to abandon the study of the aetiological role of hospital admission factors, such as age, family situation and social class. If one wishes to study factors (e.g. food, and alcohol and tobacco consumption) which are related to those mentioned above patients and controls should be made more comparable by matching them for age and social class. Lastly, by considering several types of control it is possible to assess better the bias they introduce and to some extent to prevent it. The best controls are patients with a disease of equal severity who therefore have similar admission factors.

(c) *Target population defined by community, such as a family, a profession or any other group*

Family studies might, for example, involve comparison of a sick twin with a healthy twin or a sick spouse with an unaffected spouse; such studies enable matching which may be beneficial in interpretation of results. But the possibility of bias must be considered. The same risk exists with surveys in professions; it may be supposed, for instance, that patients presenting with asthmatic disorders are less numerous in certain occupational groups, so a negative correlation could be found between risk factors and asthma.

Registers in general practice may also serve as a basis for case-control studies, but here there are different causes of bias. For example, it is likely that poorer patients seek medical advice only for serious diseases whereas the wealthy do so for mild disorders as well. Hence comparison of a seriously affected patient with a slightly affected control will create an artificial social class difference.

(d) A combination of populations

Comparisons have been made between hospital patients and samples (representative or not) of a population defined on an administrative basis. Similarly, patients from occupational communities have been compared with controls in a neighbouring administrative area. Selection bias will probably exist in this type of sampling: hospital patients often differ from controls taken from the district in which the hospital is located, both in their social class (they are often of lower social class), and in their place of residence, since the hospital's catchment area may be greater than the district from which controls are taken—the same type of bias applies in other communities.

SAMPLING METHODS

(a) Type of sampling

In case-control studies, one or more control subjects are selected for each patient. Theoretically both controls and patients must be randomized within their total groups. For example, if it is assumed that in an administrative area there are 1000 patients and 1 000 000 controls, it is possible to include 500 patients in the study (by selecting one patient out of two at random) and 500 controls (by selecting one control out of 2000 at random). But this method is often difficult, and controls are often chosen by more or less defined means which sometimes create a new source of bias.

Proper matching of controls and patients is essential to improve their comparability. The process involves the choice of one or more controls of the same sex, age, place of residence for each patient. Matching is done for each case; an example is the study of the aetiological role of oral contraceptives in myocardial infarction (Mann, Inman and Thorogood 1976): all women under the age of 50 who died of myocardial infarction in 1973 in England were traced from the files of the Registrar General. All women who died before the age of 40, one death out of two in the 40–44 age group and one death out of three in the 45–49 age group were included in the survey; the general practitioners who treated these women were questioned about the oral contraceptives prescribed and for each death one woman matched for age and conjugal status was chosen from the general practitioner's list. This study shows how the methods of randomization and matching can be combined.

Matching can also be achieved by means of stratified sampling. For example, in a survey to investigate the aetiology of premature births cases can be matched according to the mother's age, with the population broken down into homogeneous subgroups by age (e.g. 15–19, 20–24 etc). Within each five-year stratum controls equal to the number of premature infants are drawn by a random method. This method, which requires knowledge of the criterion of stratification, in this case mother's age, for the entire population, is often difficult to use.

As mentioned before methods of matching are essential in studies carried out in hospitals to eliminate the effect of hospital admission factors. But they are also useful in surveys outside hospitals: for example comparison of lung cancer patients with persons without cancer on a general population basis would demonstrate age and sex differences and lead to a number of other differences which would considerably hamper aetiological interpretation.

(b) *The size of the sample*

Decisions on sample size are particularly difficult in case-control studies in which a number of comparisons between patients and controls are made. The number of subjects required thus depends on the following factors:

1. distribution of the variable being studied in the control group (mean and variance if it is quantitative or proportion if it is a qualitative one);

2. the likely size of the difference to be found;

3. the risk α of finding a difference where there is none;

4. the risk β of missing a real difference;

5. the hypothesis of the effect of the variable, i.e. does it increase or decrease the frequency of the illness.

Using these factors the number of cases can be calculated. Detailed formulae and tables are given in Appendix 1.

(c) *Definition of patients and controls*

This involves both defining the criteria for diagnosing the disease being studied, and selecting a group of criteria resulting from definition of the population and the sample.

Criteria for diagnosis must describe the disease and, if necessary, the stage of development, and the treatment given etc. It must also be specified whether the study is to include all the cases in the population (prevalence) or just the new cases (incidence). All the aspects of accuracy, sensitivity and repeatability related to any diagnostic techniques must be considered but two factors which specifically relate to case-control studies are particularly important.

These studies are rarely based on systematic detection of sick individuals in the population group; more often it is a question of people seeking medical advice because of an illness. This can, of course, attenuate the differences expected because there may be unknown sick people in the control group.

What is more serious is the likelihood of making a diagnosis from the aetiological characteristics studied: if the wealthy seek medical advice more readily than the poor for minor symptoms of the disease studied, there is the risk of finding a relationship between social class and the disease. If smokers are subjected to more thorough investigations there is a risk of finding an aetiological relationship between tobacco and particular diseases. Included in this category of bias is the association between two diseases often observed under hospital conditions, in which case one is considered to play a role in the aetiology of the other. This association is often a result of admission (a patient is more likely to be admitted to hospital for two diseases) and the gravity of the disease (a serious disease results in more thorough examination than a mild one).

The criteria resulting from definition of the population and the sample must include all the factors considered under the headings 'Choice of Target Population' and 'Sampling Methods'. These vary considerably from study to study but it must be remembered that over-complex definition of the target population may lead to a preliminary study which is too cumbersome.

INVESTIGATIONS

Investigation into aetiological factors are often performed on the basis of data collected after diagnosis of the disease, usually by means of interview; but these investigations may take place before diagnosis.

ERRORS IN DATA

Data collected after the diagnosis of a disease are likely to contain errors of several types. For example, some result from forgetfulness: events of little importance or short duration are generally forgotten in a few days or perhaps weeks and so if an interview takes place several years later you could only expect valid information on notable or lengthy illnesses.

Other errors are related to the patient's knowledge of the field studied: medical knowledge, for instance, plays an important role if the aetiological factors sought concern previous illnesses and their treatment; general intelligence, competence in the language of the country etc. are also important. The goodwill of the patient questioned and his previous conditioning also play a part. In retrospective surveys, these errors affect comparison between patients and controls who may not reply in the same way on the questionnaire. Thus, replies to questions are affected by patients' physical state, their ideas about the aetiology of the disease and any interest they may have in the study.

The investigator also introduces error: if he knows the diagnosis he may tend to question patients more carefully than controls and to avoid asking controls certain rather delicate questions.

Everything must be done to avoid these serious errors. Whenever possible interviewing should be done before investigator and patient become aware of the diagnosis. Questions should be as objective as possible and phrased so that the investigator uses the same words when addressing both patients and controls.

Clinical or biological investigations carried out after the appearance of disease create problems of interpretation as it may be difficult to decide what results from aetiological factors and what is a consequence of the disease itself: case-control studies of the role of Type 2 herpes virus in the aetiology of carcinoma of the cervix have illustrated this. The ideal situation is when a risk factor is present before and after diagnosis.

Because of the errors described investigations must be carried out before diagnosis of disease whenever possible. The increased use of administrative, medical or opinion surveys and of data banks may enable confirmation of information which exists in the framework of a case-control study. The difficulties however are considerable; some are theoretical such as the use of data for a purpose other than originally intended and others are practical such as the problem of access to old information and linkage with current information.

NON-RESPONSE

Subjects who for some reason are not included in all or some of the investigations are also an important source of error. These non-respondents, which in case-control studies arise after diagnosis, affect comparison between patients and controls as they will probably be distributed unequally between the two groups.

The best solution is to avoid the factors which cause non-response or to carry out new investigations on all non-respondents or a representative sample selected by the usual random method. However, it may be useful to constitute this sub-sample of non-respondents quickly so all the subjects can be interviewed at the same time. For this, Dalenius (1957) suggested a method whereby the subjects present have a greater chance of being selected than do absent subjects. Thus the sub-sample of non-respondents is constituted ipso facto.

Another method, such as replacing a non-respondent by another subject similar to the non-respondent is also very difficult to perform correctly and often leads to a false sense of security and may engender a wrong result.

ANALYSIS OF RESULTS

Analysis takes place in several stages using a number of different techniques which include the following:

techniques to compare the characteristics of the patients and controls (χ^2, mean comparison);

assessment of the risk connected with the aetiological factor studied;

a study of aetiological factors allowing for other factors (partial comparisons, adjustments, multivariate analyses).

The details of these rather general techniques are illustrated in the example in Appendix 2. A brief description is given here of calculation of the relative risk because of its particular relevance to these studies.

CALCULATION OF RELATIVE RISK

If it is simply a case of analysing the association between one aetiological factor and one disease a simple test of comparison (χ^2, if a qualitative characteristic is involved), enables determination of whether the difference found between patients and controls is significant.

It may be useful to calculate the risk associated with the aetiological factor. Two examples must then be considered.

Table 1 in Appendix 2 illustrates the factors involved in a study of prevalence. Various indices have been proposed, in particular the M_1/M_0 ratio. This has been used by Hammond and Horn (1954) to measure the high mortality rate of smokers.

Using a case-control study it is possible to evaluate the proportion of subjects exposed to a risk factor among the healthy and the sick. The formulae are as follows:

$$X_0 = \frac{n_{10}}{n_{00}+n_{10}} \qquad X_1 = \frac{n_{11}}{n_{01}+n_{11}}$$

In general, the frequency of disease in a population is unknown, but it is still possible to calculate relative risk provided the disease is rare in subjects both exposed and not exposed to the risk factor. This relative risk is the M_1/M_0 ratio. The following estimation was proposed by Cornfield (1951):
$$\frac{M_1}{M_0} = \frac{N_{11}}{N_{01}} \times \frac{N_{00}}{N_{10}}$$

AN EXAMPLE OF THE ANALYSIS

This example was taken from a survey by Institut National de la Santé et de la Recherche Médicale in France (INSERM) (Schwartz et al 1966) which compared 612 male patients with angina pectoris followed-up in two hospital cardiology departments, with 612 controls of the same age and sex who had been admitted to the same hospitals after accidents at work or road accidents. The aim of this survey was to study the role of tobacco in the aetiology of coronary diseases. The analysis is further detailed in Appendix 2 but it can be summarized in three phases: first, comparing the quantity of tobacco smoked between the two groups; second, studying the role of inhalation, taking account of the quantity of tobacco smoked (Table 2 in Appendix 2) and the role of the number of cigarettes taking account of inhalation (Table 3 in Appendix 2); and third, calculation of the relative risk taking account of both inhalation and the quantity smoked (Table 4 in Appendix 2).

STRATEGY OF THE ANALYSIS

The example given is relatively simple, but often the epidemiologist has to devise a more complicated strategy for analysis. This strategy must first of all relate to the aims of the study, i.e. an investigation of causation hypotheses or the determination of risk factors. In the first case the procedure will be the successive elimination of secondary factors in order to determine the essential aetiological factor or factors which differentiate patients from controls, when all other factors are equal. The search for risk factors, on the other hand, takes into account all the factors (including those which play no aetiological role, as well as the initial symptoms) in order to specify, for instance, a forecasting formula in which each of them receives the appropriate weighting.

In case-control studies there are also a number of sampling factors likely to alter interpretation of the results:

1. If the study contains several sets of controls, it must be decided whether patients should be compared with each other to determine if any factors in the recruitment of controls produce any major differences between them.

2. If any matching is involved, it is necessary to note how this will be accounted for in the calculations.

3. If the beginning of the analysis indicates that controls and patients are not comparable in the methods used for questioning or sampling, it should be possible to introduce appropriate matching and adjustment to improve the situation.

CASE-CONTROL STUDIES IN EPIDEMIOLOGICAL RESEARCH

Case-control studies have several practical advantages; frequently they are shorter and less costly than prospective studies which means they are the most natural method available for testing hypothetical associations which clinical observation or comparisons in time and space may suggest.

However case-control studies have many limitations: some result from mistakes in sampling (particularly in hospital studies) and others from the biases created by interviewing after the appearance of a disease. It is also difficult to adapt case-control studies to biological or clinical exploration.

In addition to the limitations peculiar to case-control studies, there are the restrictions placed on any observation inferring causality. However it is still true that this type of study, if judiciously employed, constitutes a line of approach which is sometimes more effective than large scale prospective studies: recent examples of the risk of thromboembolism among women using oral contraceptives have shown this (Mann, Inman and Thorogood 1976). But when all is said and done, their appropriate and successful use simply stems from good research strategy.

APPENDIX I

DETERMINATION OF THE NUMBER OF SUBJECTS FOR A CASE-CONTROL STUDY

CALCULATION

(a) *The aetiological factor is a quantitative variable*

n_A = number of controls

n_B = number of patients

$\overline{X}_A$ = mean value of the aetiological factor in the group of controls

X_B = supposed mean value of the factor in the group of patients

Δ = the difference to be demonstrated = $\overline{X}_B - \overline{X}_A$

δ^2 = variance, which is supposed to be identical in the two groups (controls and patients)

ϵ_α = value of normal variable reduced according to the risk α ($\epsilon = 1.96$ if $\alpha = 5$ per cent)

ϵ_β = value of normal variable reduced according to the risk β ($\epsilon = 1.96$ if $\beta = 5$ per cent)

Where the sign of difference Δ is known the number of subjects required is provided by the following formula:

(1)
$$\frac{1}{n_B} + \frac{1}{n_A} \leqslant \frac{1}{(\epsilon_{2\alpha} + \epsilon_{2\beta})^2} \cdot \frac{\Delta^2}{\delta^2} \text{ (see Table 1)}$$

Where the sign of difference Δ is unknown and the number of subjects required is higher:

(2)
$$\frac{1}{n_B} + \frac{1}{n_A} \leqslant \frac{1}{(\epsilon_\alpha + \epsilon_{2\beta})^2} \cdot \frac{\Delta^2}{\delta^2} \text{ (See Table 2)}$$

(b) *The aetiological factor is a qualitative variable*

n_A = number of controls

n_B = number of patients

P_A = percentage of the aetiological factor in the group of controls

P_B = percentage of the factor in the group of patients

ϵ_α = value of normal variable reduced according to the risk α ($\epsilon = 1.96$ if $\alpha = 5$ per cent)

ϵ_β = value of normal variable reduced according to the risk β ($\epsilon = 1.96$ if $\beta = 5$ per cent)

Where the sign of difference Δ is known, the number of subjects required is provided by the following formula:

(1)
$$\frac{1}{n_B} + \frac{1}{n_A} \leqslant 4 \frac{(\text{arc sin } \sqrt{P_B} - \text{arc sin } \sqrt{P_A})^2}{(\epsilon_{2\alpha} + \epsilon_{2\beta})^2} \text{ (see Table 3)}$$

Where the sign of difference Δ is unknown the number of subjects required is higher:

(2)
$$\frac{1}{n_B} + \frac{1}{n_A} \leqslant 4 \frac{(\text{arc sin } \sqrt{P_B} - \text{arc sin } \sqrt{P_A})^2}{(\epsilon_\alpha + \epsilon_{2\beta})^2} \text{ (see Table 4)}$$

Table 1. *Number of subjects necessary per group for comparing two means (unilateral test,* $\alpha = \beta = 5\%$ *and* $n_A = n_B$. (*Source: Schwartz, Flamant and Lellouch 1970*)

$\Delta/\delta \times 100$	0	1	2	3	4	5	6	7	8	9
10	2164.6	1788.9	1503.2	1280.8	1104.4	962.0	845.6	749.0	668.1	599.6
20	541.1	490.8	447.2	409.2	375.8*	346.4	320.2	296.9	276.1	257.4
30	240.5	225.2	211.4	198.8	187.3	176.7	167.0	158.1	149.9	142.3
40	135.3	128.8	122.7	117.1	111.8	106.9	102.3	98.0	94.0	90.2
50	86.6	83.2	80.0	77.1	74.2	71.6	69.0	66.6	64.3	62.2
60	60.1	58.2	56.3	54.5	52.8	51.2	49.7	48.2	46.8	45.5
70	44.2	42.9	41.8	40.6	39.5	38.5	37.5	36.5	35.6	34.7
80	33.8	33.0	32.2	31.4	30.7	30.0	29.3	28.6	28.0	27.3
90	26.7	26.1	25.6	25.0	24.5	24.0	23.5	23.0	22.5	22.1
100	21.6	21.2	20.8	20.4	20.0	19.6	19.3	18.9	18.6	18.2
110	17.9	17.6	17.3	17.0	16.7	16.4	16.1	15.8	15.5	15.3
120	15.0	14.8	14.5	14.3	14.1	13.8	13.6	13.4	13.2	13.0
130	12.8	12.6	12.4	12.2	12.1	11.9	11.7	11.5	1.4	11.2
140	11.0	10.9	10.7	10.6	10.4	10.3	10.2	10.0	9.9	9.7

* Example: for $\Delta/\delta \times 100 = 25$, at the intersection of line 20 and column 5, n = 346.4. Condition of application: the final value for n must be fairly large (at least 30)

Table 2. *Number of subjects per group for comparing two means (bilateral test* $\alpha = \beta = 5\%$ *and* $n_A = n_B$). (*Source: Schwartz, Flamant and Lellouch 1970*)

$\Delta/\delta \times 100$	0	1	2	3	4	5	6	7	8	9
10	2599.1	2148.0	1805.0	1538.0	1326.1	1155.2	1015.3	899.3	802.2	720.0
20	649.8	589.4	537.0	491.3	451.2*	415.9	384.5	356.5	331.5	309.0
30	288.8	270.5	253.8	238.7	224.8	212.2	200.5	189.9	180.0	170.9
40	162.4	154.6	147.3	140.6	134.2	128.3	122.8	117.7	112.8	108.2
50	104.0	99.9	96.1	92.5	89.1	85.9	82.9	80.0	77.3	74.7
60	72.2	69.8	67.6	65.5	63.5	61.5	59.7	57.9	56.2	54.6
70	53.0	51.6	50.1	48.8	47.5	46.2	45.0	43.8	42.7	41.6
80	40.6	39.6	38.7	37.7	36.8	36.0	35.1	34.3	33.6	32.8
90	32.1	31.4	30.7	30.0	29.4	28.8	28.2	27.6	27.1	26.5
100	26.0	25.5	25.0	24.5	24.0	23.6	23.1	22.7	22.3	21.9
110	21.5	21.1	20.7	20.4	20.0	19.6	19.3	19.0	18.7	18.4
120	18.0	17.7	17.5	17.2	16.9	16.6	16.4	16.1	15.9	15.6
130	15.4	15.1	14.9	14.7	14.5	14.3	14.0	13.8	13.6	13.5
140	13.3	13.1	12.9	12.7	12.5	12.4	12.2	12.0	11.9	11.7

* Example: for $\Delta/\delta \times 100 = 25$, at the intersection of line 20 and column 5, n = 415.9. Condition of application: the final value for n must be fairly large (at least 30)

Table 3. *Number of subjects necessary per group for comparing two percentages* (*unilateral test,* $\alpha = \beta = 5\%$ *and* $n_A = n_B$). (*Source: Schwartz, Flamant and Lellouch 1970*)

*P' \ *P	5%	10%	15%	20%	25%	30%	35%	40%	45%	50%
5%	—	584.3	182.5	95.4	60.9	43.2	32.6	25.7	20.8	17.3
10%	584.3	—	938.2	268.8	132.8	81.4	55.8	41.1	31.6	25.2
15%	182.5	938.2	—	1244.4	341.1	163.5	97.7	65.7	47.5	36.0
20%	95.4	268.8	1244.4	—	1505.6	402.2	188.6	110.7	73.3	52.3
25%	60.9	132.8	341.1	1505.6	—	1723.0	451.7	208.5	120.7	79.0
30%	43.2	81.4	163.5	402.2	1723.0	—	1896.9	490.1	223.3	127.8
35%	32.6	55.8	97.7	188.6	451.7	1896.9	—	2027.1	517.5	233.2
40%	25.7	41.1	65.7	110.7	208.5	490.1	2027.1	—	2113.9	533.9
45%	20.8	31.6	47.5	73.3	120.7	223.3	517.5	2113.9	—	2157.3
50%	17.3	25.2	36.0	52.3	79.0	127.8	233.2	533.9	2157.3	—
55%	14.6	20.5	28.2	39.1	55.6	82.7	132.1	238.1	539.4	2157.3
60%	12.4	17.0	22.7	30.3	41.2	57.6	84.5	133.5	238.1	533.9
65%	10.7	14.3	18.6	24.1	31.6	42.2	58.3	84.5	132.1	233.2
70%	9.2	12.1	15.4	19.4	24.8	32.0	42.2	57.6	82.7	127.8
75%	8.0	10.3	12.8	15.9	19.7	24.8	31.6	41.2	55.6	79.0
80%	7.0	8.8	10.8	13.1	15.9	19.4	24.1	30.3	39.1	52.3
85%	6.0	7.5	9.0	10.8	12.8	15.4	18.6	22.7	28.2	36.0
90%	5.2	6.3	7.5	8.8	10.3	12.1	14.3	17.0	20.5	25.2
95%	4.3	5.2	6.0	7.0	8.0	9.2	10.7	12.4	14.6	17.3

*P and P' are the percentages in the two groups to be compared. One must be known or estimated from which the other can be deduced using the real difference (P−P') that it is required to detect with α and β fixed at 5 per cent, and the knowledge of the percentages, or the region in which their values lie ($\simeq$ P+P'/2). If both exceed 50 per cent their complements may be used.

Condition of application: the final value for n must be fairly large (at least 20)

Table 4. *Number of subjects necessary per group for comparing two percentages (bilateral test* $\alpha = \beta = 5\%$ *and* $n_A = n_B$). (*Source: Schwartz, Flamant and Lellouch 1970*).

*P' \ *P	5%	10%	15%	20%	25%	30%	35%	40%	45%	50%
5%	—	701.6	219.2	114.6	73.1	51.8	39.1	30.8	25.0	20.7
10%	701.6	—	1126.5	322.7	159.5	97.7	67.0	49.3	38.0	30.2
15%	219.2	1126.5	—	1494.0	409.9	196.3	117.3	78.9	57.0	43.2
20%	114.6	322.7	1494.0	—	1807.9	482.9	226.4	133.0	88.0	62.8
25%	73.1	159.5	409.9	1807.9	—	2069.0	542.4	250.3	145.0	94.8
30%	51.8	97.7	196.3	482.9	2069.0	—	2277.6	588.5	268.1	153.5
35%	39.1	67.0	117.3	226.4	542.4	2277.6	—	2434.0	621.3	280.0
40%	30.8	49.3	78.9	133.0	250.3	588.5	2434.0	—	2538.3	641.0
45%	25.0	38.0	57.0	88.0	145.0	268.1	621.3	2538.3	—	2590.4
50%	20.7	30.2	43.2	62.8	94.8	153.5	280.0	641.0	2590.4	—
55%	17.5	24.6	33.9	47.0	66.8	99.3	158.6	285.9	647.6	2590.4
60%	14.9	20.4	27.2	36.4	49.5	69.2	101.5	160.3	285.9	641.0
65%	12.8	17.1	22.3	28.9	37.9	50.7	70.0	101.5	158.6	280.0
70%	11.1	14.5	18.4	23.4	29.7	38.4	50.7	69.2	99.3	153.5
75%	9.6	12.3	15.4	19.1	23.7	29.7	37.9	49.5	66.8	94.8
80%	8.4	10.5	12.9	15.7	19.1	23.4	28.9	36.4	47.0	62.8
85%	7.2	9.0	10.8	12.9	15.4	18.4	22.3	27.2	33.9	43.2
90%	6.2	7.6	9.0	10.5	12.3	14.5	17.1	20.4	24.6	30.2
95%	5.2	6.2	7.2	8.4	9.6	11.1	12.8	14.9	17.5	20.7

*P and P' are the percentages in the two groups to be compared. One must be known or estimated from which the other can be deduced using the real difference $(P-P')$ that it is required to detect with α and β fixed at 5 per cent, and the knowledge of the percentages, or the region in which their values lie ($\simeq P+P'/2$). If both exceed 50 per cent their complements may be used.

Condition of application: the final value for n must be fairly large (at least 20)

APPENDIX 2

EXAMPLE OF THE METHOD OF ANALYSIS

In this example 612 male patients presenting with angina pectoris are compared to 612 controls (Schwartz et al 1966).

The first phase of the analysis consisted of comparing the quantity of tobacco smoked in each of the two groups; no difference was found in the amount of pipe smoking; but the patients smoked more cigarettes (18.6 versus 15.5; $P = 10 - 5$) and inhaled more often (59 per cent versus 45 per cent; $P = 10 - 5$).

The second phase of the analysis was to study the role of inhalation, taking into account the quantity of tobacco smoked (Table 2) and the role of the number of cigarettes, taking inhalation into account (Table 3). Partial comparisons showed that patients inhaled more often than controls, irrespective of the number of cigarettes smoked. Among subjects who did not inhale, patients and controls smoked similar quantities of tobacco; on the other hand, among those who did inhale, patients smoked more than controls: consequently it seems that the number of cigarettes played a role only if the subjects inhaled.

These observations enabled calculation of the relative risk taking account of both inhalation and the amount smoked (Table 4). Inhalation more than doubles the risk from the amount smoked.

The technique of partial comparisons illustrated by Tables 3 and 4 is generally used in case-control studies to make patients and controls more comparable. It is based on a simple statistical test (χ^2, mean comparison). It is also possible to use one method of adjustment (Rumeau-Rouquette and Schwartz 1970) which enables account to be taken of all the results in a single overall test. In Table 2 such a test would account for the four factors studied.

Table 1. *Distribution of subjects within the population. The figures placed in the boxes represent the subjects (Source: Rouquette and Schwartz 1970)*

	Patients		
Exposed	No	Yes	% Patients
No	N_{00}	N_{01}	$M_0 = N_{01}/(N_{00}+N_{01})$
Yes	N_{10}	N_{11}	$M_1 = N_{11}/(N_{10}+N_{11})$

Table 2. *Aetiological role of inhalation taking account of the number of cigarettes smoked (Source: Schwartz et al. 1966)*

Number of cigarettes/day	Groups	Number of cases	% of subjects inhaling	Significance
1–9	Patients	47	40	$P > 0.05$
	Controls	52	25	
10–19	Patients	67	70	$P = 0.01$
	Controls	102	48	
20–29	Patients	98	81	$P = 0.01$
	Controls	87	62	
30+	Patients	59	88	$P = 0.001$
	Controls	29	55	

Table 3. *Aetiological role of the number of cigarettes, taking account of inhalation* (*Source: Schwartz et al 1966*)

Inhalation	Groups	Number of cases	Number of cigarettes/day	Significance
No	Patients	74	14.8	P > 0.05
	Controls	138	14.2	
Yes	Patients	197	22.6	P = 0.001
	Controls	132	18.6	

Table 4. *Relative risk; the risk for non-smokers was 1.0* (*Source: Schwartz 1966*)

	Number of cigarettes per day				
Inhalation	1–9	10–19	20–29	30+	Total
No	0.8	0.4	0.7	0.6	0.6
Yes	1.7	1.1	1.7	3.8	1.7
Total	1.0	0.8	1.3	2.4	

REFERENCES

Berkson, J. (1946) Limitation of the application of fourfold table analysis to hospital data. *Biometrics Bulletin 2*, 47.

Berkson, J. (1958) Smoking and lung cancer: some observations on two recent reports. *Journal of the American Statistical Association, 53*, 28

Butler, N. R. & Alberman, D. (1969) *Perinatal Problems.* The second report of the 1958 British Perinatal Mortality Survey. London: Churchill Livingstone

Cornfield, J. (1951) A method of estimating comparative rates from clinical data. Application to cancer of the lung, breast and cervix. *Journal of the National Cancer Institute, 2*, 1269

Dalenius, T. (1957) *Sampling in Sweden.* Stockholm: Almqvist and Wiksell

Hammond, E. C. & Horn, D. (1954) The relationship between human smoking habits and death rate. *Journal of the American Medical Association, 155*, 13

Mann, J. I., Inman, W. H. W. & Thorogood, M. (1976) Oral contraception use in older women and fatal myocardial infarction. *British Medical Journal, 2*, 445

Rumeau-Rouquette, C., Bréart, G., Deniel, M., Hennequin, J. F. & du Mazaubrun, C. (1976) La notion de risque en périnatalogie. Résultats d'enquêtes épidémiologiques. *Revue d'Epidémiologie et de Santé Publique, 24*, 253

Rumeau-Rouquette, C. & Schwartz, D. (1970) *Méthodes en Epidémiologie.* Paris: Flammarion

Schwartz, D., Flamant, R. & Lellouch, J. (1970) *L'Essaie Thérapeutique Chez l'Homme*. Paris: Flammarion
Schwartz, D., Lellouch, J., Anguera, G., Beaumont, K. L. & Lenègre, J. (1966) Tobacco and other factors in the etiology of ischemic heart disease in man. *Journal of Chronic Diseases, 19,* 35
Stewart, A., Webb, J. & Hewitt, D. (1958) A survey of childhood malignancies. *British Medical Journal, 1,* 1495
Tuyns, A. J., Jensen, O. M. & Pequignot, G. (1977) Le choix difficile d'un bon groupe de témoins dans une enquête rétrospective. *Revue d'Epidémiologie et de Santé Publique, 25,* 67

SUGGESTED TEXTS FOR BACKGROUND READING

Holland, W. W. (1970) *Data Handling in Epidemiology*. London: Oxford University Press
Jenicek, M. (1976) *Introduction à l'Epidémiologie*. Paris: Maloine
Kessler, I. J. & Levin, M. L. (1970) *The Community as an Epidemiologic Laboratory*. A casebook of community studies. Baltimore: Johns Hopkins University Press
Lilienfeld, A. M. (1976) *Foundations of Epidemiology*. New York: Oxford University Press
MacMahon, B. & Pugh, T. F. (1970) *Epidemiology: Principles and Methods*. Boston: Little Brown

CHAPTER 6

The Application of Retrospective Studies to Health Care Research

John Ashley

The retrospective, or case-control, method of enquiry which is commonly used in epidemiological investigations of aetiology can be modified for use in the study of problems associated with the need for health services or the delivery of medical care, particularly when there is a need to interpret different patterns of utilization. In designing such studies it is not appropriate to consider 'cases' and 'controls' as such, but instead comparable groups with, say, differing levels of utilization, are selected. There are certain practical considerations not applicable to retrospective studies of aetiology, but the simplicity of this method makes it eminently suitable for use at a local level. It may also form part of a general research strategy for investigation of more extensive problems.

DEFINITIONS

In chapter 5 Rumeau-Rouquette has described the application of retrospective, or case-control, studies to aetiological epidemiological research. Such studies may be defined by their ability to meet three essential criteria, as follows:

their objective is to test hypotheses;
their method involves a comparison of two predetermined groups;
and their approach is retrospective.

Some studies which seek to estimate prevalence may also involve, in part, a comparison between two or more groups of subjects. However in such comparisons the definition of such groups is generally made a posteriori whereas in typical case-control studies the comparative groups are defined a priori when the study is designed.

Each of the essential criteria can be subject to a degree of modification particularly when the method is adapted to apply in other fields, such as that concerned with the need for health services or the delivery of medical care.

THE NEED FOR HYPOTHESES

It is generally of practical as well as of theoretical importance to formulate a specific hypothesis for testing before embarking on a case-control study. In this way the study can be designed so that it will achieve a specified objective and also the sample size and the amount of data collected on each subject can often be reduced. Nevertheless in aetiological research it is also quite common to use the case-control method to explore a range of predisposing or risk factors. Such a procedure is equally relevant to studies of health care problems, particularly those directed at interpreting different patterns of utilization of services. Furthermore, as many health care problems have multiple causes it is often desirable to design studies to cover a range of factors and hence be in a position to determine the relative influence of each.

COMPARATIVE GROUPS

It has been suggested (MacMahon and Pugh 1970) that the term *case-comparison* study might be more appropriate than the term *case-control* study because an investigation of this type does not usually incorporate the same kind of control situation as that used in an experimental study. It is clear that in the study of aetiology the only rational basis of selection of comparative groups is to choose those with the disease and those who are unaffected. Yet it would be equally legitimate to compare two groups both of whom had the disease, but with differing degrees of severity. Indeed sometimes the planning, and frequently the analysis, of traditional case-control studies is extended to three or more groups in this way.

There are health care situations in which it is possible to identify an 'affected' and an 'unaffected' group. For example, the characteristics of those who make use of preventive services may be compared with those who do not. Nevertheless it is more usual to use the case-control method to make comparative studies of utilization between, for example, institutions, clinics, administrative areas or diagnostic groups, or alternative treatment regimes. In such situations it is clear that it is not practicable to consider the groups under study either as 'cases' or 'controls'.

Because of the method of analysis used and because they do not fall into any of the other classifications of epidemiological study it is appropriate to include the methods and problems of such investigations in this chapter.

RETROSPECTIVE APPROACH

Accepting that the two criteria of objective and design can be interpreted somewhat liberally allows consideration, in this category, of a wide range of comparative studies, provided that they meet the third criterion in that they are retrospective. Often there is a lack of clarity in the way 'retrospective' is defined, but it is generally acknowledged that studies of this nature entail the collection of information about past events, obtaining such data from patients or subjects by interview, carried out during or after the event, or by the review of written records which are independent of the observer.

THE SCOPE OF CASE-CONTROL STUDIES IN HEALTH CARE RESEARCH

In aetiological studies the choice between the case-control and the prospective cohort approach is influenced both by the extent of existing clinical or statistical knowledge of the condition being investigated and by its incidence. In a prospective study a large number of subjects is often required so that the investigation will yield enough cases of the disease to obtain significant results: for such a study to be practical the implication is that the disease has to have a relatively high incidence; similar principles apply to studies of health care and its procedures. A prospective cohort study of a health care situation is only economically viable if there is a substantial likelihood of its members being subjected to the particular procedure under investigation. Thus there is considerable scope for the alternative case-control method which is not restricted in this way. Nevertheless studies using this method are not applicable to all aspects in the field of medical care research which covers investigations into a wide range of aspects of the preventive and curative services. The aspects of these services particularly include:

the determination of their need;

their pattern of use;

the evaluation of their effect.

One further factor is of particular importance. Studies of health care are frequently designed in a comprehensive way in response to a defined problem. In consequence it is common to find that, within a single investigation, there are elements of both retrospective and prospective studies and from them it is often possible, for example, to also determine the 'incidence' or 'prevalence' of an aspect of health care.

THE DETERMINATION OF NEED

The need for any service encompasses not only the extent to which that service is required by the average general population, but also how it might have to be modified for a particular sex, social class or geographical area of residence or treatment. In consequence comparative studies of need are frequently carried out. However these are, in effect, modified surveys of incidence or prevalence, and case-control studies as such can only be of limited use in the estimation of need. Nevertheless comparative studies can shed some light on specific needs. In an investigation into the need for intensive nursing care in a teaching hospital (Garrett et al 1966) a sample of cases assessed as requiring such care were compared with a random sample of all patients discharged from the same hospital during the period of the study. This served to identify the diagnostic categories and operations likely to given rise to patients who would need the special facilities for intensive nursing care which the general results of the study indicated were necessary.

THE PATTERN OF USE

In contrast, the case-control method is particularly important for determining the significance of external factors which affect service utilization. This method is particularly relevant to this type of problem because of its simplicity and the rapidity with which it is possible to obtain an answer, both to general and local queries.

GENERAL FACTORS INFLUENCING USE

There are many factors of a general nature which can affect the use of services and much light can be shed on the various influences by a comparative study of matched users of a service in an area of high 'take-up' with those in an area where the 'take-up' is low. For example, it has recently been shown that there is considerable variation in the amount of night visiting undertaken by general practitioners (Buxton, Klein and Sayers 1977). This study correlated night consultation rates for a range of administrative areas with several other characteristics of the areas concerned, but because of the limited amount of routine data available only the most basic suggestions can be made about possible causes of the variation. This observation suggests, as a next step, a study which identifies matched groups of users of the service in areas of high and low utilization and compares the characteristics of each group. This example further illustrates why case-control studies of the utilization of health services frequently compare situations of high and low use, rather than situations of 'use' and 'non-use'. In this case there would be considerable theoretical and practical difficulties in identifying a group of patients who did not consult general practitioners at night.

Querido (1963) has described a similar situation in a study which compared the psychological background of a sample of children who were admitted to hospital several times with a control group who were only admitted once. Although this study suggested that certain psychological traits in the families concerned contributed to the repeated admissions, it was regrettable that no comparison was possible with an 'ideal' control group composed of children who had never been admitted to hospital. It was decided not to attempt to obtain such a group because of the intimate nature of the interview that was carried out to obtain the data required.

Another classical comparative study explored differences in the pattern of utilization of outpatient services between two groups of hospitals (Chamberlain 1966). In each hospital group the records of over 800 consecutive new outpatients seen within a calendar year were reviewed, and this demonstrated considerable differences in the demographic and social characteristics between those attending the two groups of hospitals.

LOCAL USE OF THE CASE-CONTROL METHOD

The simplicity of elementary comparative studies, which are the most fundamental form of case-control studies make them eminently suitable for use at a local level. This is particularly relevant because of a further difference which is often found between medical care and epidemiological studies. Epidemiological studies are usually directed at determining the relevance of certain defined factors in the aetiology of a specific condition or syndrome, so that once a comprehensive study has been carried out there is generally little need to repeat it. Many medical care problems may only exist in a particular locality or population because of the particular combination of external factors. Similarly the same problem may be present in two different localities, but the underlying reasons may be quite different. Let us consider patients who have a prolonged stay in hospital for a specified surgical procedure. Surgical beds and the facilities associated with them, such as operating theatres, are often provided on a scale which assumes a rapid turnover of patients, however for a variety of reasons some patients will inevitably remain in the beds for longer than usual. On some occasions this is for medical reasons, for example if complications develop. At other times a longer stay may be for 'administrative' reasons; there may, for example, be a lack of operating theatre time, or delay in performing investigatory procedures (Querido 1963). There may also be social factors that preclude the patient's discharge.

Thus it may well be necessary to carry out similar studies in different areas to show the same basic problem in order to identify local reasons and hence suggest a local solution. Murphy (1977) carried out one such study applying the case-control method to data obtained from a special census of all the 265 occupied orthopaedic and general surgical beds in an administrative area and which identified a group of 80 patients with a stay, hitherto, of more than 28 days. Within this group there were 43 patients whose condition, as assessed by the nursing staff, no longer required them to be in an acute ward. The characteristics of this subgroup of cases, defined as 'social long-stay' were compared with those of a control subgroup comprising the remaining 37 long-stay cases each of which had a definable medical or nursing need for care in an acute ward. Even with these small numbers it was possible to discern differences between the two subgroups in their age and sex structure, and also in their previous length of stay and diagnostic pattern. In consequence recommendations were made regarding improvement in cooperative measures to help alleviate the problem. Nevertheless, in this study, restricted research resources prevented what might have been an equally interesting and important comparison between comparable groups of long-stay and short-stay cases.

THE EVALUATION OF SERVICES

Case-control studies can be used to evaluate medical care services, nevertheless it must be acknowledged that there is greater merit in assessing the comparative effectiveness of two treatments or services by means of a prospective study, if possible in the form of a controlled trial. If, however, the urgency of the study requires the collection of retrospective data, then the establishment and subsequent comparison of two or more retrospective cohorts is usually the preferred method of approach. Cohort studies of this nature are often carried out in order to evaluate a medical care procedure by, for example, determining the relative incidence of complications after two alternative surgical operations. Such an approach, although it has a retrospective element is not a retrospective study, as defined. Nevertheless when carried out in this manner such studies frequently enable the case-control method to be applied to the data in such a way as to demonstrate the influence certain factors have on which patients present for the procedure in question. This may be illustrated from a study primarily directed at the determination of the incidence of depression after hysterectomy (Richards 1973). This study compared events of depressive illness in a cohort of 200 patients who had a hysterectomy with a control group who had other operations. In order to assess the effectiveness of the matching process, it was also important to determine the number of events of such illness in each group in the period before operation. This procedure is effectively also a simple case-control study of the role of previous depressive illness on the presentation for hysterectomy, and in the event revealed that in the hysterectomy group there was a higher incidence of previous depression (19 per cent) than in the control group (4 per cent).

It is also possible for a simple study to be concerned both with aetiological and health care aspects of the same condition, and a variation of this is the study aimed at one aspect which reveals important information about the other. To return to Rumeau-Rouquette's example in Chapter 5 of the study designed to investigate the aetiology of cervical cancer: the interpretation of the findings from an aetiological point of view was that the control group which consisted of patients with benign conditions was considered unsatisfactory. If, however, these controls who were of lower social class with bigger families came from the same hospital and were expected to be as representative as the cancer cases, this finding might provide an interesting insight into selection procedures in the hospital concerned.

SOME PRACTICAL CONSIDERATIONS

Many of the practical considerations specified in connection with the design, method and analysis of case-control studies in aetiology also apply when medical care problems are studied, but in addition further practical difficulties are encountered which affect:
1. choice of venue for a study;
2. availability of sampling frames;
3. selection of cases;
4. matching.

CHOICE OF VENUE
The geographical location of many medical care studies is often restricted by the need to find an environment where there will be sufficient co-

operation and goodwill to allow projects to reach a satisfactory conclusion. Thus there is a tendency to select locations for a study on this basis, rather than at random. This often means that the places chosen may not be entirely typical or they may not represent the full range of variation of the health care parameter under study.

For example, if a study is to be carried out to determine the use of general practice it may not be possible, because of their workload, to obtain sufficient cooperation from single-handed practitioners. Much depends on the persuasive skill of the investigator if it is imperative that a particular environment is investigated, or if the areas or institutions to be studied have been selected, say, to form a stratified random sample.

AVAILABILITY OF SAMPLING FRAMES AND SELECTION OF CASES

These two considerations are frequently interrelated, since selection of cases may be restricted to those recorded on available lists or registers: such lists, for example of attenders at clinics or of admissions to hospital, are easily sampled. Often, however there are no such lists available at the appropriate time: this particularly applies when the investigation is set up to study cases of a specific diagnosis, although sometimes a retrospective index which will help in assessing the validity of the study may be subsequently available. In such circumstances, sampling frames may have to be specially constructed; the attendant problems are illustrated in a study of health care concerned with hospital practice. As before, although this study was initially designed as a prospective study it has important retrospective elements which proved crucial in interpretation of the problem at which it was directed. It sought to identify the factors influencing case-fatality rates of patients treated in hospital for hyperplasia of the prostate (Ashley, Howlett and Morris 1971).

CASE SELECTION IN HYPERPLASIA OF THE PROSTATE

This study stemmed from the observation, first noted by Lee, Morrison and Morris (1957) that there were lower case-fatality rates for a variety of common surgical conditions in patients treated in undergraduate and postgraduate teaching hospitals in England and Wales than in those treated in other hospitals, which at the time were managed by Regional Hospital Boards. These differences, which were identified in routine hospital data, from the *Hospital In-Patient Enquiry*, were found for such conditions as appendicitis, peptic ulcer, and hyperplasia of the prostate and persisted after simple standardization for age, sex and source of admission (e.g. emergency or otherwise). Subsequently these findings were repeated using further data which included a range of medical as well as surgical conditions (Lipworth, Lee and Morris 1963).

From the start of these investigations a number of explanations were suggested, which centred round two major themes: the first was that of selection of less complicated cases by the teaching hospitals; the second, which appeared to be the more likely, was that there was superior care in the teaching hospitals where there were more doctors, nurses and other resources. Although some of the conditions did not entail surgical intervention it was commonly thought that much of the effect of superior care would be channelled into post-operative management of surgical cases. It thus seemed appropriate, when it was decided to carry out an in-depth study to elucidate the situation, that hyperplasia of the prostate should be chosen as a representative condition: it involves surgical management in elderly men for whom deficiencies in the standard of post-operative care might be crucial in terms of life or death.

In view of the most favoured hypothesis it was tempting to restrict the study to a prospective one which examined the mortality and complications of prostatectomy which was found to be the treatment carried out on virtually all cases admitted. Operating theatre registers could provide an easily accessible and readily available list of these cases and so this approach would have presented few problems. However it was considered important to review all cases of the disease whether they were operated upon or not, and thus to be in a position to compare the case material presenting at each hospital. It was anticipated that this would enable further exploration of the factors related to possible selection of cases by teaching hospitals: thus, it was necessary to identify patients likely to have this condition soon after they were admitted to hospital and so a variety of information sources were used, but the mainstay was regular enquiries among ward staff.

Whereas other and subsequent enquiries elicited a few missed cases eventually diagnosed as having the condition, over a quarter of those included at first eventually had to be excluded because they failed to satisfy the necessary diagnostic criteria. Even so, it was often difficult to convey the qualifications for entry to the study to frequently changing ward staff. In particular, many found it difficult to understand that a study of outcome carried out on surgical wards should include patients not destined for operation.

These decisions on methodology proved correct as the study was able to show that many of the differences in case-fatality rates between hospitals could be attributed to case selection. Furthermore, cases on whom operations were not performed, and who would have been neglected if the original design had been adopted, were crucial in determining overall mortality from the condition.

Difficulties are not always experienced in deriving a suitable sampling frame from existing hospital nursing records. It was found to be practicable in the study of intensive nursing care needs, described earlier (Garrett et al 1966) and in an investigation into the possible adverse effects on female schizophrenic patients of a prolonged stay in a mental hospital (Wing and Brown 1970).

This latter study was also of a prospective nature but included a retrospective element which attempted to correlate the social environment in three hospitals with clinical differences between their patients. The three hospitals were deliberately selected because they had markedly different social conditions and administrative policies, but within them patients were randomly selected. The matron of each hospital supplied a list of female schizophrenic patients aged under 60, who had been inpatients for more than two years. From these lists the intention was to draw a random sample of 120 cases in each hospital, but in one hospital only 73 cases satisfied the predetermined criteria. One hundred cases were required to satisfy the study design, and the extra twenty were to act as 'spares' for the next stage, which was a review of case notes for each of the hundred cases: this was carried out in order to check that the patient concerned fitted defined diagnostic criteria, and to replace in the sample any that failed to do so; five such replacements were necessary. In addition a random sample of all case notes in each hospital was reviewed to ensure that an adequate yield had been obtained by the method adopted; a few extra cases were found.

The effectiveness of the method of ascertainment in this study certainly reflects the accurate knowledge among senior nursing staff in psychiatric hospitals. There were also a number of other advantages which would not necessarily apply to other similar studies. All the patients had been in hospital for considerable time and so were likely to have extensive records expressing medical opinion about their diagnosis. Schizophrenia is a diagnosis which is unlikely to change over time, and this chronicity also made it possible for sufficient time to elapse between drawing the sample and interviewing the patients, to allow reporting by a senior well-qualified person with long-standing knowledge of the patients and their conditions.

MATCHING

In any investigation it must be decided to what extent particular factors should be excluded from the beginning of the study or perhaps subsequently eliminated by methods of standardization or other similar procedures. In health care studies there is a real risk that such exclusions may eliminate the very differences, for example in the case-mix, that are most significant in solving the problem: thus most such studies do not attempt to restrict the scope of relevant variables. Similarly it is not common to match sampled cases initially on an individual basis: the usual practice is to match the groups on as broad a basis as possible and to carry out more detailed group or individual matching on subsamples during analysis. Even at this stage however, there are certain limitations in the use of matched selected subsamples as the basis for comparative analysis: it may be found that certain categories cannot be matched in all the situations under review and thus have to be excluded from the analysis, however important they may seem.

One further point that should be remembered when carrying out the analysis is, as was shown in the hyperplasia of prostate study, the need to show conclusively that the data obtained do indeed demonstrate the problem under consideration; this requirement affects health care studies rather more than it does aetiological investigations.

CONCLUSION

Health care research is an applied science and the data with which it is associated are frequently less clear cut than those used in the epidemiology of causation. Similarly many of the techniques used have to be modified to meet the needs and idiosyncrasies of the subject. This applies to the case-control study, just as it does to studies of incidence and prevalence, or to randomized controlled trials. Nevertheless the very nature of problems related to the use or delivery of health care implies that studies are often designed which incorporate elements of various methods and these could increasingly include retrospective investigations of a case-control nature.

REFERENCES

Ashley, J. S. A., Howlett, A. & Morris, J. N. (1971) Case-fatality of hyperplasia of the prostate in two teaching and three regional-board hospitals. *Lancet, 2,* 1308

Buxton, M. J., Klein, R. E. & Sayers, J. (1977) Variations in GP night visiting rates: medical organisation and consumer demand. *British Medical Journal, 1,* 827

Chamberlain, J. (1966) Studies of hospital out-patient services: two non-teaching hospitals in south-east England. In *Problems and Progress in Medical Care* (Second Series) McLachlan, G. (ed). London: Oxford University Press

Garrett, S. A. G., Stephenson, R. L., Holland, W. W. & Roth, I. Z. (1966) The need for intensive nursing care. *British Journal of Preventive & Social Medicine, 20,* 34

Lee, J. A. H., Morrison, S. L. & Morris, J. N. (1957) Fatality from three common surgical conditions in teaching and non-teaching hospitals. *Lancet, 2,* 785

Lipworth, L., Lee, J. A. H. & Morris, J. N. (1963) Case-fatality in teaching and non-teaching hospitals 1956–59. *Medical Care, 1,* 71

MacMahon, B. & Pugh, T. P. F. (1970) *Epidemiology.* Boston: Little Brown

Murphy, F. W. (1977) Blocked beds. *British Medical Journal, 1,* 1395

Querido, A (1963) *The Efficiency of Medical Care.* Leiden: Stenfert Kroese

Richards, D. H. (1973) Depression after hysterectomy. *Lancet, 2,* 430

Wing, J. K. & Brown, G. W. (1970) *Institutionalism and Schizophrenia.* Cambridge: Cambridge University Press

SUGGESTED TEXTS FOR BACKGROUND READING

Morris, J. N. (1975) *Uses of Epidemiology.* Edinburgh: Churchill Livingstone

Logan, R. F. L., Ashley, J. S. A., Klein, R. E. & Robson, D. M. (1972) *Dynamics of Medical Care.* London: London School of Hygiene & Tropical Medicine

SECTION 4
PREVALENCE STUDIES

CHAPTER 7

Prevalence Studies

André Meheus

Prevalence figures estimate the number of events, i.e. diseases in a given population over a fixed period. Prevalence studies are used to describe the distribution of disease or other variables in a population, particularly chronic conditions and disability. Such descriptive information on health status is useful for health care planning.

Prevalence data is more readily available than incidence data but it gives no insight into aetiology of disease. In planning a prevalence study there must be: a clear objective; specified population; correct sampling if required; standardized examination techniques and careful recording. Particular attention to non-response is essential.

A number of examples are described: the health interview and examination surveys of the United Kingdom and the United States; prevalence studies of chronic respiratory disease in the UK and the Netherlands; and estimation of the prevalence of byssinosis in the flax industry in Belgium.

DEFINITIONS

Prevalence or cross-sectional studies are based on a single examination of a population at a particular time. Such studies will either lead to calculation of the prevalence rate,[1] i.e. the proportion of the subjects with illness or disability, or they will give prevalence or frequency distributions of qualitative and quantitative variables. This cross-section can be compared to a fixed picture of the state of health of the population at a given time (point-prevalence).

After a prevalence study, the population can be followed for a certain period to detect new cases (i.e. the incidence rate). This type of study is referred to as an incidence or longitudinal study (see Section 5).

The sum of the point-prevalence and incidence rates for a given

[1] Strictly speaking, the term 'prevalence' and not 'prevalence rate' should be used, as prevalence is not a rate but a proportion.

disease, gives the period-prevalence rate. For example the number of patients treated for tuberculosis in the county of Antwerp in 1975 gives the numerator of a period-prevalence rate, because it includes the cases that are being treated at the beginning of 1975 and the new cases whose treatment begins during 1975.

Because of the importance of distinguishing between existing cases and new ones the two fundamental frequency measures of (point) prevalence and incidence are normally used separately.

The above definition of prevalence study implies that such a study is carried out at 'a particular point in time'. In practice, it is more accurate to say 'over the period of time necessary to carry out the investigation'.

In some instances the prevalence study may last for some time; as a result it is sometimes wrongly concluded that an incidence figure is being sought. For example, in a study involving 500 pregnant women in 1971, a gonorrhoea infection was searched for at their first pre-natal consultation and an 'incidence' of one per cent was determined (Spence 1973). Although this study lasted for a year it should not be referred to as 'incidence'. Because each pregnant woman was only examined once and therefore existing cases were being diagnosed at a particular moment, the 'prevalence' of gonorrhoea was obtained (Meheus 1974).

OBJECTIVES

Prevalence studies have a number of objectives:

description of the prevalence and the distribution of a disease or other variables in a population;

detecting associations between certain variables and the illness prevalence in order to postulate hypotheses concerning the aetiology of the disease;

acting as the initial stage of an analytic (case-control or cohort study) or of an experimental or an intervention study.

Because of the method used in prevalence studies there is often the by-product of some individual screening.

ADVANTAGES AND DISADVANTAGES OF PREVALENCE STUDIES

Prevalence studies do not normally last as long as routine data collection systems and longitudinal studies and as a result they cost less, involve fewer personnel and provide data far quicker.

Such studies are particularly useful in planning various parts of the health care structure (e.g. buildings, manpower, etc.) because they provide valuable descriptive information about the state of health of the general population and of specific subgroups. Quantifying a population's state of health is the very basis for determining health needs. Certain studies provide such information on the non-institutionalized population, for example the United Kingdom General Household Survey and the United States National Health Interview and Examination Surveys which will be discussed later.

Prevalence studies also give descriptive information about various qualitative characteristics of members of a population, for example the possible risk factors for certain diseases.

As a result of this primary prevention activities can be made more efficient (e.g. health education) and in the long run they can also be evaluated.

Prevalence studies may reveal for example, that many of those suffering from a particular disease do not seek medical care or are not provided with such care. As a result these studies give a more accurate picture of the actual disease pattern than do hospital data. Hospital data are inherently biased because of selection of more serious cases for hospital admission.

The finding that in any population a considerable amount of illness has not been treated or diagnosed has led to a new form of health care known as 'screening'. This is based on the assumption that the state of health of a population can be improved as a result of early diagnosis and treatment (particularly for chronic diseases). Screening of the population can be compared with a cross-sectional study, the aim of which is not determination of the magnitude and distribution of a disease in the population but rather the early detection of high risk groups and treatment of cases.

One of the prerequisites for introduction of screening is a sufficiently high prevalence of the disease. Screening as a form of health care remains somewhat controversial because in relation to most diseases its effectiveness and efficiency has not been sufficiently demonstrated (Wilson and Jungner 1968; Cochrane 1972; *The Lancet* 1974; Sackett and Holland 1975; South-East London Screening Study Group 1977). Sackett and Holland point out that the definitions, objectives and characteristics of screening, case-finding, diagnosis and epidemiological survey must be clearly distinguished.

Prevalence is a good frequency measure for relatively long-term conditions including permanent disability or chronic illnesses. It enables determination of the 'burden' of these conditions on the community (see Chapter 8 for a description of the use of prevalence studies in estimating the health needs and demands of older sections of the population).

Prevalence is not a good frequency measure for acute illness or acute episodes in chronic diseases. This is because prevalence (P) is a function of the incidence (I) of the disease (number of new cases per time unit) and the duration (d) of the disease, as shown in the following formula:

$$P \sim I \times d$$

Hence, diseases of short duration such as acute appendicitis have a low prevalence in the population. The duration of a disease depends on the time that elapses before recovery or death.

Prevalence is also dependent on possible selective migration out of or into the population. In assessing or comparing location, time or section of population in terms of prevalence rates of disease, information about recovery, case-fatality and migration out of the population of the cases in question is necessary.

Most chronic diseases cannot be cured but it is possible to prolong the survival period (for example, for chronic respiratory diseases, cancers and mental illness). The effect of this is that whereas incidence may be stationary, prevalence is increasing.

Prevalence studies can be used to formulate hypotheses about the possible aetiological role of a certain variable in the origin of a disease, based on finding an association between the prevalence and the particular variable. For example, the prevalence of coronary heart disease (CHD) in a representative sample of the population can be investigated in relation to various personal characteristics such as age, sex, body build, smoking and eating habits, blood pressure and serum cholesterol, in order to find certain positive or negative associations. However, such data do not allow conclusions about causality of certain factors to be made because both personal characteristics (the possible causes) and the disease (the effect) are being measured at the same time. In order to discover something about causality, the causes must precede the effect.

Possible aetiological associations are better illustrated by the observation that certain characteristics lead to a higher risk of disease. Since the incidence rate is a direct measure of the disease risk (prevalence rate is also determined by the duration of the disease) it follows that the incidence study is ideal for aetiological research.

Tables 1 and 2, which are based on prevalence and incidence rates of CHD in the Framingham study, illustrate the ambiguity in interpretation of prevalence figures.

Table 1. *Prevalence of coronary heart disease (CHD) at initial examination among 4469 persons 30–62 years of age, Framingham study (Source: Mausner and Bahn 1974)*

Age (years)	Males			Females			Male/female ratio of prevalence rates
	Number examined	Number with CHD	Rate per 1000	Number examined	Number with CHD	Rate per 1000	
30–44	1083	5	5	1317	7	5	1.0
45–62	941	43	46	1128	21	19	2.4
Total	2024	48		2445	28		

Table 2. *Incidence of coronary heart disease (CHD) over an eight-year period among 4995 persons 30–59 years of age, free of CHD at initial examination. (Source: Mausner and Bahn 1974)*

Age (years)	Males			Females			Male/female ratio of incidence rates
	Number examined	Number with CHD	Rate per 1000	Number examined	Number with CHD	Rate per 1000	
30–39	825	20	24.2	1036	1	1.0	24.2
40–49	770	51	66.3	955	19	19.9	3.3
50–59	617	81	131.3	792	53	66.9	2.0
Total	2212	152		2783	73		

In the younger age groups, the prevalence rate of CHD is the same for both men and women (5 per 1000; Table 1). Incidence rates, however, indicate that the risk of getting CHD is more than 20 times higher in young men than in young women (Table 2). The explanation for this is the different duration of CHD in young men and young women: in young men CHD takes the form of myocardial infarction and sudden death, whereas in young women the illness generally lasts longer and may often result in anginal complaints. These tables also show that between men and women the difference in coronary heart disease risk decreases sharply with age.

METHODOLOGY

OBJECTIVES

The objective of a prevalence study should be clearly defined in advance, i.e. the questions to be answered and how precise the answers should be. There should be some idea of the time required to complete the study and the financial and logistic resources needed (manpower, material). The literature should be consulted with special attention devoted to information about reproducibility and validity of the research techniques to be used.

DEFINING THE POPULATION

The study attempts to determine the number of cases of disease in a population. This population is defined as a group of people who share a particular natural characteristic such as residence, profession, sex, or race.

The choice of population depends on the objective of the study and is usually fairly straightforward. Examples are a population of schoolchildren in a well-defined geographical area, a factory population, members of a particular profession or a population of pregnant women.

Once the population is defined one must decide whether the whole group should be examined or only part (a sample) of it. In the latter case the nature and size of the sample have to be defined. The choice between examining a whole population or only a sample depends on factors such as the size and attainability of the population and the complexity of the research method.

Smaller populations such as factory populations or professions are often studied as a whole, whereas in larger populations it is only practical to study a sample.

SAMPLING

Before applying sampling techniques, the sample size must be estimated approximately. The sample must be large enough to contain a substantial number of people with the disease, so sample size must be larger in diseases with lower prevalence.

Sample size also depends on the degree of precision required, which is determined by the sampling error. In a prevalence study (Barker and Rose 1976) the sampling error is measured by the standard error of a proportion:

$$SE = \sqrt{\frac{p(100-p)}{n}}$$

p = percentage of affected people
n = number in sample.

On about 95 per cent of occasions the sample estimate of prevalence will fall within two standard errors (± 2 SE) of the population prevalence.

If we have some idea of the prevalence of the condition (p) and we indicate the precision wanted for the estimate (determined by ± 2 SE), from the formula, the sample size n can be calculated. Because sampling error is proportional to the square root of sample size, doubling of sample size increases precision only by a factor of 1.4.

For continuously distributed variables, such as weight, blood pressure, or serum cholesterol the sampling error is given by the standard error of the mean (SEM):

$$SEM = \sqrt{\frac{s^2}{n}}$$

s = between-subject standard deviation
n = number of subjects.

The estimated sample mean falls with 95 per cent confidence limits within 2 SEM of the population mean. If the investigator indicated the precision wanted for the estimated mean (SEM) and as the between-subject standard deviation is generally known from previous studies, the number of subjects can be calculated. For serum cholesterol for instance a 95 per cent confidence interval of 10 mg per cent requires examination of approximately 250 subjects.

This probability calculation is only meaningful if samples are selected by random methods. If the sample is based on subjects who volunteer for the study, it is difficult to make generalizations as volunteers are generally a highly selected group (depending on the subject of the study, there is over-representation of healthy or diseased individuals). The principle of random sampling is that each sampling unit (subject, household or factory) has an equal chance of being included in the sample.

When a population list has been established a number is allocated to each individual, and a sample of the required size is selected using a table of random numbers (single random sample).

Another method is selection of every 'nth' person on the list, which yields a systematic sample. Instead of sampling individual units (individual, household or village), a group or cluster of these units can be sampled, and then each unit in the cluster is completely surveyed—this saves field work time and reduces cost. This method is known as cluster sampling.

A stratified random sample divides the population into distinct subgroups or strata according to an important characteristic such as age, sex or socio-economic status, and a random sample is drawn from each stratum. The investigator can select the same proportion of subjects from each stratum or he can take a larger proportion from strata with less subjects, in order to obtain enough subjects with that characteristic.

When large populations are studied, it is more practicable to draw the required sample in a series of stages i.e. 'multi-stage sampling'. For instance, to study tuberculin sensitivity in schoolchildren in a geographical area, first a random sample of schools is selected from a list of schools in the area, secondly a simple random sample of children is taken in each school.[2]

DATA COLLECTION AND ANALYSIS

Procedures of history-taking and examination must be standardized to limit observer variability, so standardized records must be designed (questionnaires for interview or self-administration, and standard examination forms). Comprehensive publications describing standardized procedure are available, for instance, for cardiovascular and nutritional diseases (Rose and Blackburn 1968; Jelliffe 1966).

For most types of analysis data must be expressed in a numerical form; precoded records can be used (each answer is identified by a code number), or alternatively space is left on the records to write down the code. The coded data are transferred to 80 column punched cards. These punched cards can be retrieved by a mechanical 'counter-sorter' to provide simple tabulations, but in larger surveys they are analysed by computer. This is rarely a rapid task as the computer must be programmed for the analysis; however, more and more standard programs are available in computer libraries.

During coding and transcribing in data preparation for analysing errors can easily occur, so thorough checking of both coding and punching is necessary.

Analysis of cross-sectional studies is possible without sophisticated machinery by listing subjects and their characteristics and making tables using a tallying method.

RESPONSE RATE

All efforts to extract a random sample from the population are useless if the response rate is too low (preferably it should be over 80 per cent). Therefore it is vital that a high proportion of subjects in the sample are prepared to cooperate. This can be expected when:

the design of the study is clearly explained and the cooperation of responsible people within the group is ensured;

---

[2] Sampling methodology is described in many excellent textbooks (e.g. Yates 1960; Desabie 1966; Stuart 1968; Som 1973).

the participants feel that they will benefit from the investigation;

there is no financial loss involved;

the research procedure does not cause fear or discomfort among the participants.

Non-respondents are generally not a random subgroup: they probably include too many diseased or too many healthy people depending on the subject of study. The bias caused as a result of non-response has to be estimated. Some of the methods for doing this are:

to check whether prevalence of the condition in those who have cooperated only after repeated calls differs from that in immediate respondents;

to try to examine a subsample of non-respondents;

to compare examined and non-examined groups in relation to particular characteristics such as sex, age, profession or absenteeism data;

to check the reasons for not participating.

Eylenbosch et al (1973) determined the prevalence of cardiovascular diseases in a random sample of 500 post office workers aged 20–64 years in the province of Oost-Vlaanderen (Belgium). The prevalences for the age group 40–59 only are summarized in Table 3. The response rate was 83 per cent.

To get an indication of possible selection bias, the group of non-participants is studied for different items, such as sickness, absenteeism data, motive for non-participation, and age distribution. For example, in Table 4 the age distribution of examined and non-examined groups of the random sample is given; if we consider only the age groups 40–59 (see Table 3), the examined group is not biased for age. (For the whole age range of the sample the 30–39 age group and the 60–64 age group are respectively over- and under-represented.)

EXAMPLES OF PREVALENCE STUDIES

HEALTH INTERVIEW AND EXAMINATION SURVEYS

Health interview surveys, such as the US National Health Interview Survey (US HIS) and the health section of the UK General Household Survey (UK GHS), are a particular type of prevalence study. Conducted on a national scale, a random sample of households is selected and by trained interviewers data are collected on prevalence of illness, disability and restriction of activity, on incidence of acute illness, on the use of health and related social services, on attitudes towards the health services, and on self-medication.

Table 3. *Prevalence (%) of cardiovascular symptoms and of ECG abnormalities in a random sample of postal workers (age group 40–59 years; N = 219)*

	Prevalence %
Angina	7.8
Possible infarction	3.6
ECG-probable ischaemia	3.6
ECG-possible ischaemia	10.9

Table 4. *Age distribution (%) of examined and non-examined group in a random sample of 500 postal workers*

Age group (years)	Examined (N = 406) (%)	Non-examined (N = 94) (%)
20–29	9.3	9.9
30–39	30.5	16.5
40–49	34.4	36.3
50–59	19.4	21.7
60–64	6.1	15.4
All ages	99.7	99.8

Table 5. *Prevalence of (a) reporting of limiting long-standing illness in 1971 in Great Britain and (b) reporting of chronic limitation of activity in 1972 in the United States, for different age groups (Sources: (a) Office of Population Censuses and Surveys 1973, (b) United States Department of Health, Education and Welfare 1974)*

Age group (years)	(a) UK GHS 1971 prevalence %	(b) US HIS 1972 prevalence %
< 15 (UK GHS)/< 17 (US HIS)	4.7	3.0
15–44 (UK GHS)/17–44 (US HIS)	9.0	8.3
45–64	24.9	21.1
⩾ 65	43.5	43.2
Total	15.9	12.7

In Table 5, the prevalence of chronic limitation of activity in 1972 in different age groups in the US and the UK is given. For both countries there is a comparable increase of chronic sickness with age and the prevalence rates found are very similar.

A recent conference on National Health Survey Systems in the European Community recommended collaborative action especially in health

Table 6. *Prevalence rates in the United States 1963–1965 for colour vision defi-ciencies among children 6–11 years of age by race and sex (Source: US Dept Health, Education and Welfare 1972*

Race and sex	Estimated number of children affected	Rate per 100 children
Both sexes		
Total	902 000	3.80
Boys		
Total	839 000	6.95
White	773 000	7.44
Negro	66 000	4.04
Girls		
Total	63 000	0.53
White	50 000	0.50
Negro	13 000	0.76

interview surveys (Armitage 1977) and discussed the possibility of having comparable data, particularly on disease prevalence and health service utilization, for many European Countries.

In the US a continuous health examination survey has been established: it is based on physical examinations, clinical and laboratory tests and various other measurements of national samples of the population. This Health Examination Survey gives estimates of prevalence of specific diseases in the US and the frequency distributions of physical, physio-logical and psychological characteristics of that population.

As an example, in Table 6, prevalence rates of colour vision defects in US children are given. Sex differences in prevalence of colour vision defects are apparent; boys are 13 times more likely to have a defect than girls.

PREVALENCE STUDIES OF CHRONIC LUNG DISEASE

Lambert and Reid (1970) determined in a prevalence study the amount of chronic non-specific lung disease (CNSLD) in the population of Great Britain. This is described according to various characteristics such as age, sex, place of residence, degree of air pollution in the environment and smoking habits. For this purpose, a random sample of the whole population in the age group 35–69 was questioned using a postal ques-tionnaire. The estimated response rate was 74 per cent, which is con-sidered by some to be high for a postal survey. Respondents were representative in terms of age, sex and urban-rural distribution, but the

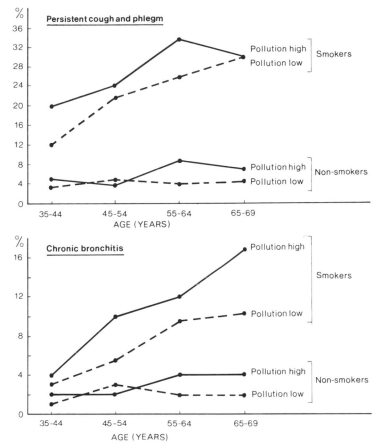

Figure 1. Prevalence of 'persistent cough and phlegm' and 'chronic bronchitis' in relation to smoking and air pollution in different age groups (Source: Lambert & Reid 1970)

authors indicate that there might be a bias in social class with a high proportion of members of social classes IV and V. The association between smoking habits, air pollution, age and prevalence of respiratory symptoms is summarized in Figure 1. These data show that the prevalence of respiratory symptoms in non-smokers varies little according to the degree of pollution, except in older age groups.

Generally speaking smokers show a much higher prevalence of respiratory symptoms, and in this group there is a distinct difference in prevalence between polluted and non-polluted areas. This is already

Table 7. *Prevalence rate of respiratory symptoms in males in various surveys* (*Source: Van der Lende 1969*)

	Netherlands			Great Britain	United States of America	Czecho-slovakia
	Meppel 40–59 N = 1709 (%)	Vlagt-wedde 40–59 N = 902 (%)	Vlaar-dingen 40–59 N = 569 (%)	London 40–59 N = 250 (%)	East coast towns 40–59 N = 625 (%)	Brno 40–64 N = 2736 (%)
Q. 5 Persistent cough	21.3	23.5	27.4	39.2	30.9	40.2
Q. 10 Persistent phlegm	14.9	14.3	24.4	40.0	31.8	36.7
Q. 14a Dyspnoea gr. 2 or more	(14.1)	28.3	26.8	59.2	40.6	—
Q. 14b Dyspnoea gr. 3 or more	4.5	7.5	5.2	9.2	—	13.2
Q. 15a Ever wheezed	30.6	32.3	28.1	—	—	—
Q. 15c Wheeze most days and/or nights	7.7	10.1	7.3	18.0	9.1	—
Q. 22 (16) Asthmatic attacks	4.3	4.3	1.9	1.2	4.0	6.4
Q. 5+10 Persistent cough and persistent phlegm	12.5	12.0	16.6	32.8	23.5	—
Q. 12 One or more chest illnesses	—	8.9	11.7	18.8	21.6	—
Q. 5+10+12 Persistent cough and persistent phlegm and one or more chest illnesses	—	4.0	3.3	10.8	6.9	—

shown in younger age groups and the difference is even more apparent for complaints of 'chronic bronchitis'. From these data one can hypothesise that smoking cigarettes and to a lesser degree air pollution, might be aetiological factors in the development of chronic respiratory diseases. Likewise one can postulate that a synergic effect between smoking and air pollution is highly probable. The importance of such findings is that they can form the basis for primary prevention activities.

Van der Lende (1969) completed several prevalence studies of CNSLD in the Netherlands, using a standardized methodology which enabled

Table 8. *Number of cases of byssinosis and CNSLD according to departments in two flax industries*

Departments	Byssinosis	CNSLD	No respiratory complaints	Total
Weaving mill	18	14	10	42
Shearing mill	2	3	1	6
Preparatory				
Weaving mill I	0	6	10	16
Weaving mill II	4	1	2	7
Maintenance	0	2	2	4
Ready-made shop	0	9	43	52
Finishing	0	11	3	14
General services	1	5	5	11
Administration	0	1	3	4
Total	25	52	79	156

comparison with similar studies in other countries. Table 7 shows a comparison of the prevalence of respiratory symptoms in a number of studies, based on the UK Medical Research Council questionnaire, slightly modified in some cases.

The prevalence of persistent cough and persistent phlegm is lower in the Dutch areas, although Vlaardingen which is an urban polluted area has a prevalence figure which does not differ much from the figures of other countries. The explanation of the observed differences in prevalence is difficult; therefore such factors as smoking habits, air pollution, and occupational exposure to dust must be considered.

PREVALENCE STUDY OF BYSSINOSIS

Byssinosis in the flax industry was not a recognized occupational disease in Belgium but because of a possible alteration in the law it was necessary to determine the 'magnitude' of this disease in the flax industry (Vuylsteek et al 1967). All workers in two flax weaving mills were examined and the prevalence of byssinosis and CNSLD was obtained on the basis of a standardized questionnaire—the results are shown in Table 8.

The prevalence of byssinosis was 25/156 (16 per cent), but it appeared that the disease was more prevalent among workers involved in the early stage of flax production, particularly in the weaving mill. This department had 42 workers out of which 18 (43 per cent) suffered from byssinosis.

The 42 workers who were apparently heavily exposed to the risk of byssinosis were a 'survivor-population' of all the workers who had worked in those particular departments; it was also important to determine the prevalence of the disease among workers who had left those departments.

In the period from 1955 till 1965, 192 workers had left these departments; 142 were available for examination and the prevalence of byssinosis was found to be 56 per cent in this group.

On the basis of this descriptive study, the authors could both determine the 'magnitude' of the byssinosis problem in the flax industry and also indicate those departments where workers are at higher risk.

REFERENCES

Armitage, P. (1977) *National health survey systems in the European Community—Final Report*. Proceedings of a conference held in Brussels on 6–8 October 1975 (EUR 5747e) Luxembourg: Commission of the European Communities

Barker, D. J. P. & Rose, G. (1976) *Epidemiology in Medical Practice*. Edinburgh: Churchill Livingstone

Cochrane, A. L. (1972) *Effectiveness and Efficiency: Random Reflections on Health Services*. London: Nuffield Hospitals Trust

Desabie, G. (1966) *Théorie et Pratique des Sondages*. Paris: Dunot

Eylenbosch, W., Doumit, J., Meheus, A., De Meyere, M. & Vuylsteek, K. (1973) Prevalentie van cardiovasculaire aandoeningen bij postbeambten. *Tijdschrift voor Sociale Geneeskunde, 51*, 542

Jelliffe, D. B. (1966) *The Assessment of the Nutritional Status of the Community*. Geneva: World Health Organization

Lambert, P. M. & Reid, D. D. (1970) Smoking, air pollution, and bronchitis in Britain. *Lancet, 1*, 853

Lancet (1974) Screening for disease. *Lancet, 2*

Mausner, J. S. & Bahn, A. K. (1974) *Epidemiology: An Introductory Text*. Philadelphia: W. B. Saunders

Meheus, A. (1974) Incidence and prevalence (letter). *Obstetrics and Gynecology, 44*, 313

Office of Population Censuses and Surveys (1973) *The General Household Survey—Introductory Report*. London: Her Majesty's Stationery Office

Sackett, D. L. & Holland, W. W. (1975) Controversy in the detection of disease. *Lancet, 2*, 357

Som, R. K. (1973) *A Manual of Sampling Techniques*. London: Heinemann

South-east London Screening Study Group (1977) A controlled trial of multiphasic screening in middle age: results of the south-east London screening study. *International Journal of Epidemiology, 6*, 357

Spence, M. R. (1973) Gonorrhea in an military prenatal population. *Obstetrics and Gynecology, 42*, 223

Rose, G. A. & Blackburn, H. (1968) *Cardiovascular Survey Methods*. Geneva: World Health Organization

Stuart, A. (1968) *Basic Ideas of Scientific Sampling*. London: Griffin
United States Department of Health, Education and Welfare (1972) *Color Vision Deficiencies in Children, United States*. Vital and Health Statistics, Series 11, Number 118
United States Department of Health, Education and Welfare (1974) *Limitation of Activity and Mobility due to Chronic Conditions, United States—1972*. Vital and Health Statistics, Series 10, Number 96
Van Der Lende, R. (1969) *Epidemiology of Chronic Non-Specific Lung Disease (Chronic Bronchitis)*. Assen: Van Gorcum
Vuylsteek, K., Van Ganse, W., De Sweemer, C., Eylenbosch, W., Stevens, J., Debusscher, P. & Van Cauteren, G. (1967) Byssinosis: epidemiologische studie in de vlasnijverheid. *Acta Tuberculosea et Pneumoligica Belgica, 58*, 487
Wilson, J. M. G. & Jungner, G. (1968) *Principles and Practice of Screening for Disease*. Geneva: World Health Organization
Yates, F. (1960) *Sampling Methods for Censuses and Surveys*. London: Griffin

SUGGESTED TEXTS FOR BACKGROUND READING

Barker, D. J. P. & Rose, G. (1976) *Epidemiology in Medical Practice*. Edinburgh: Churchill Livingstone
Rose, G. A. & Blackburn, H. (1968) *Cardiovascular Survey Methods*. Geneva: World Health Organization
Mausner, J. S. & Bahn, A. K. (1974) *Epidemiology: an introductory text*. Philadelphia: W. B. Saunders
Desabie, G. (1966) *Théorie et pratique des Sondages*. Paris: Dunot

CHAPTER 8

Prevalence Studies of Long-term Illness

Robert J. van Zonneveld

Prevalence studies are particularly useful for establishing health care needs of the elderly and chronic sick population. Several prevalence studies of disease and disability in the elderly population of the Netherlands are described.

A major survey was undertaken in 1952 to 'measure' the needs of the elderly for hospital care, nursing home care, residential home care, and medical and social care for those living at home, in a random sample of 3000 elderly in a large city. In 1962 the Ministry of Social Affairs and Public Health requested prevalence studies to 'measure' the need for services among the chronic sick aged 40 years and over. This study was performed in three phases: (1) a self-administered questionnaire sent to 10000 city dwellers and 10000 people of the same age group, living in a number of rural municipalities in one province; (2) an inquiry to appropriate family doctors in order to gather their opinions on the various needs; and (3) examination and interview by the same physician of the chronic ill or disabled, indicated by the previous two phases, to obtain both an objective and a subjective insight into specific needs and demands.

Finally there is a short description of a nationwide longitudinal study of the health of old people and on general aspects of their health care using information from their family doctor.

INTRODUCTION

Prevalence is the number of a particular phenomena existing in a population at a particular time. It may refer either to the number of people with a defined characteristic, e.g. of a certain height, or with a particular disease in which case prevalence describes the amount of disease in a population. Prevalence may also refer to the amount of a specific disability in a population and also to the increased risk of a certain disease or invalidity. Prevalence can be considered to be the *balance* of the bank account with incidence (see Chapter 9) on the *credit* side and death or recovery on the *debit* side.

PREVALENCE STUDIES OF THE CHRONIC SICK AND ELDERLY

Prevalence studies are particularly useful for the ageing population where chronic disorders occur more often. These chronic disorders demand more, and more varied, health and social care provision. In industrialized countries the proportion of aged people in the population is continually increasing. In future prevalence studies will become more essential for determining their health care needs. For example, for deciding what inpatient facilities are required (e.g. geriatric wards in hospitals, and nursing homes for physically and mentally sick aged) as well as what community services (e.g. domiciliary help, district health centres, and meals on wheels) are required. With the increasing dominance of chronic ailments in the pattern of disease and disability in industrialized countries the value of prevalence studies lies not so much in determining the causes of chronic diseases and disability (although they may contribute to that purpose) but in determining the most appropriate methods of care.

Prevalence studies, as well as cohort studies, are useful in gerontological research. By study of certain personal and environmental factors they can often be used to distinguish between the true symptoms of ageing, the degenerative diseases which may be prevented or at least treated in the early stages, and the effects of external factors such as cigarette smoking (Morris 1975). As a result prevalence studies are important for *secondary prevention*, which is the early detection and treatment of disease, particularly at the pre-clinical phase of a chronic disease before symptoms appear and result in the patient seeking medical attention.

The use of prevalence studies in estimating the risk factors in relation to chronic disorders and the early symptoms of these disorders is discussed in more detail in Chapter 7.

Prevalence studies also play an important role in the *tertiary prevention* of chronic diseases and ageing symptoms, i.e. the prevention of further deterioration, of complications, of invalidity and subsequent dependence, or of relapse after initial improvement. They determine the number and type of facilities for patients at various stages of dependence.

We cannot acquire a complete picture of the burden on society of chronic diseases and disorders of old age, without determining the prevalence of the incurable sick and permanently disabled.

It is clear that in order to make reasonable estimates of the need for various social and health care facilities, a single study in a certain part of the country is insufficient. Prevalence studies, for example to determine the need for nursing home beds, should take place in various locations because of the likelihood of local differences (apart from differences in the age-sex structure of the population which can be statistically accounted for)—for example, relationships between generations (whether or not younger people are willing to nurse sick parents within the home), philosophical outlook, religious denomination, socio-economic factors, degree of urbanization, existence of facilities, climate, geographical factors (access and availability of facilities, local policy, etc).

It is also necessary to repeat prevalence studies after certain periods in order to check need for provisions; this could change as a result of both new ideas about the most appropriate type of care (e.g. it is now thought that moderately fit aged persons should remain in their own homes as long as is medically and socially justified instead of being moved to residential homes), and because as more advanced diagnostic and therapeutic methods are developed changes in mortality, morbidity and disability patterns occur.

These and other factors mean that from time to time it is necessary to check if the facilities available are still in accordance with the needs of both the population and of those who provide treatment and care.

PREVALENCE STUDIES OF THE ELDERLY IN THE
NETHERLANDS

Study of Facilities for the Elderly in Groningen (van Zonneveld 1954)

In the fifties a number of residential homes[1] and nursing homes[2] were built in the Netherlands. A few of these institutions already existed, but it was felt that many more were needed. To provide further information

---

[1] In the Netherlands a 'residential home' is a home for people over 65 years. (In Dutch it is a 'verzorgingstehuis' or care providing home.) It provides accommodation for the elderly who cannot wholly or can only inadequately perform their household duties.

[2] In the Netherlands a nursing home is like a small simple hospital with between 100 and 200 beds. Medical treatment, rehabilitation, nursing, and terminal care are provided over a long period or permanently. There are over 300 such homes with a total of 42 000 beds.

about the facilities required the author, assisted by 70 medical students (all nearly qualified), carried out a random survey among 3000 elderly people (65 years and older) who, in 1952, comprised one-quarter of the elderly population of the town of Groningen. This was a descriptive study of a random sample of the population stratified by age with relatively more people examined from the older age groups. Participants were asked a number of questions and had a simple examination. Only 36 refused to cooperate giving a low refusal rate (1.2 per cent).

The objective of the survey was to gather quantitative information at a particular time about the functioning and disorders in the important organs and in other physiological systems; and about methods of adjusting to defects in order to perform important daily tasks. From the results some attempt was made to divide old people examined into groups according to their health status and according to socio-medical facilities considered to be the most suitable for them. The survey also included a memory test. Thus, the study was aimed at determing the prevalence of a number of symptoms and so the numbers of aged who required various categories of assistance.

Before the survey a pilot study of approximately 200 elderly people was carried out to test the questionnaire (which was mostly pre-coded) and method of approach and to determine the reaction to be expected from participants. A letter explaining the purpose of the survey including a request for cooperation was sent to the people before the visits took place and they were also informed of the time of the visit. The interviewers were personally instructed and their findings discussed after each visit: the information was then computerized.

Some of the findings from this prevalence study are described here. About 40 per cent of those examined had been under treatment by a physician in the three months before the study. In the older age groups no more men or women were feeling 'less well' than in the younger age groups. However significantly more women were complaining about their health. There was no significant difference between numbers complaining about their health in the higher and lower social classes. There were fewer complaints about health among men still working in the higher social classes than among those still working in the lower classes or among those who were no longer working.

Complaints about hearing were not so common as about seeing and most occurred in the oldest age group: more men complained about hearing than women. Men of 75 years and older in the lower social classes who had stopped work some years previously had more trouble

Table 1. *Appropriate socio-medical provision for the elderly (Source: van Zonneveld 1954)*

Age	At home and independent		At home with simple help		Residential home (home for the aged)		Long-stay annex (nursing home)		Hospital– geriatric department		Total	
	No.	(%)	No.	(%)	No.	(%)	No.	(%)	No.	(%)	No.	(%)
Men												
65–69	217	(48.2)	201	(44.7)	25	(5.6)	7	(1.5)	0	(0)	450	(100)
70–74	155	(38.6)	197	(49.0)	41	(10.2)	8	(2.0)	1	(0.2)	402	(100)
75–79	105	(29.9)	178	(50.7)	56	(16.0)	9	(2.6)	3	(0.8)	351	(100)
80+	33	(11.0)	133	(44.3)	104	(34.7)	27	(9.0)	3	(1.0)	300	(100)
Women												
65–69	308	(68.4)	103	(22.9)	30	(6.7)	7	(1.6)	2	(0.4)	450	(100)
70–74	215	(54.0)	119	(29.9)	50	(12.5)	13	(3.3)	1	(0.3)	398	(100)
75–79	114	(32.6)	145	(41.5)	76	(21.8)	12	(3.4)	2	(0.7)	349	(100)
80+	45	(15.0)	88	(29.3)	133	(44.3)	33	(11.0)	1	(0.4)	300	(100)

with their hearing than those in the higher social classes who had stopped work some years before. Hearing aids were rarely used and if they were little or no benefit was gained from them. In the oldest age groups hearing aids were used significantly more often but in this context there was no statistically significant difference between the sexes.

Between the two extreme age groups there was a significant difference in the results of the memory test: the younger group scored better. In the youngest group men scored significantly better than women but this sex difference was not present in the oldest group. In the higher social classes the median of results obtained were higher.

Only a few men and women had difficulties with washing and dressing, apart from in the oldest age group where 10 per cent of the men and 20 per cent of the women could not adequately perform these functions. Conditions affecting the arms and legs, and weakness were the reasons most often given. Ascending and descending stairs, caused problems for many (about 40 per cent of women and 25 per cent of men). The principal reasons given were: shortness of breath, conditions affecting the legs and dizziness.

Participants were also asked their opinion on living in old people's homes: approximately two-thirds said they were not in favour of them but women in the older age groups were more in favour while there was no significant change of opinion with increased age in men. In both the youngest and oldest age group more women than men were in favour of such institutions. Between married and unmarried (or no longer married) people no differences in opinion were found.

Considering the data for every age group in the town of Groningen, it was found that to accommodate all those who should be living in some kind of institution (without taking account of personal wishes or financial circumstances) for every 1000 people over 64 years there should be: 153 beds in old people's homes, 34 in nursing homes (including a number in special homes for the mentally infirm), and 4.3 in general hospitals. These figures are very similar to those calculated for the total elderly population of the Netherlands in 1952. More details are given in Table 1. Since then of course many circumstances have changed: for example there is now greater emphasis placed on care in the community and consequently the need for institutional care, particularly in residential homes, has decreased.

Study on the Need for Provisions for the Chronic Sick (van Zonneveld 1965/1966; Fennis 1973)
In the early sixties the Ministry of Social Affairs and Public Health in the Netherlands requested the author, then working at the Netherlands Institute of Preventive Medicine in Leiden, to carry out a survey of facilities required for the chronic sick. After the planning, setting up and carrying out the first stage, Fennis took over the study operation and analysis of the data from which the following description is derived.

Investigations were carried out into the prevalence of chronic diseases and disability of at least four weeks' duration, among people aged 40 and over; the resulting need for institutional and community facilities for these patients was calculated. The investigations took place in Leiden, a city of 100000 inhabitants, and in 10 municipalities of the Province of Friesland (Frisia) which included rural areas and urbanized rural areas.

The people investigated were selected at random from the population registers. In Leiden those selected represented a quarter of the population aged 40 or over and in Friesland they represented one-fifth of the population of the same age.

The surveys were carried out in three phases:

1. Firstly a partly retrospective mail survey with the aid of a *questionnaire* with answers mostly pre-coded. The response rate was about 90 per cent. Of the 10 per cent of non-respondents in Leiden one third were later interviewed. Their results did not differ significantly on a number of variables from respondents.

2. Secondly an *inquiry* among general practitioners in the population

surveyed. This was partly to check on the questionnaire and partly to assess the provisions the general practitioner considered necessary for their patients; it was done by direct contact (structured interview) in Leiden and by letter in Friesland.

3. Finally there was an *examination* of handicapped patients in their homes or institutions by the investigating physician. Only a few people refused this examination.

Only the data from the group aged over 65 years were used because, in relation to calculation of facilities needed the age group of 40–65 years produced almost negligible numbers. It would have been better therefore, if relatively more of the aged, and especially the very old, had been included in the random sample, as in the earlier survey of the elderly by van Zonneveld (1954).

It appears (Fennis 1973) that three factors have to some extent affected the validity of the findings:

1. sex differences in subjective assessment of the duration of illnesses;

2. mortality and prolonged hospitalization;

3. and the selection of random samples of controls (healthy people and an intermediate group of people who were not very healthy but not chronically ill either).

The two morbidity surveys covered almost 5000 aged people and taken together they reflect the national situation at the time reasonably well.

The results for people over 65 in Friesland can be summarized as follows: over 12 per cent of the men (with only minor changes occurring with age) and between 10 and 20 per cent of the women (increasing with age) suffered from chronic disorders. In order of frequency these were caused by: diseases of the respiratory, circulatory and digestive tracts, and disorders of the central nervous system. These conditions account for 55 per cent of all the chronic diseases found. It seems that during the sixties the pattern of disease among the aged has not changed much because the disease pattern found in the survey is dominated by chronic disorders illustrating that there has been little change in prevalence even with the emphasis placed on preventive techniques by health services.

In Leiden, about 8 per cent of the male and 10 per cent of the female population over 65 suffered from disabling disorders which were mainly caused by diseases of the central nervous system, cardiovascular diseases and disorders of the locomotor system. These three disorders accounted for 75–80 per cent of all disabling conditions.

The total need for institutional and community services for the elderly is 19 per cent in Leiden and 26 per cent in Friesland, half of which is for the *very* old (80+) who require 60 per cent of facilities. Of the aged between 6 and 7 per cent are suitable for admission to a residential home, half of those suitable are the very elderly. There is increasing need with age for admission to a nursing home: for both sexes this ranges from 1 per cent to between 7 and 9 per cent. In Leiden nearly 2 per cent and in Friesland nearly 3 per cent of the elderly required admission to a nursing home because of mental, as well as combined physical and mental, limitations. There are more elderly women who suffer severe mental impairment than there are men.

In relation to admission to nursing and residential homes, more women than men have to be admitted not only in absolute numbers (because there are more elderly women than men), but also relatively for each age group.

According to both surveys 60 per cent of the elderly who depend on institutional services should be admitted to a residential home; 20 per cent to a nursing home for physically handicapped and 20 per cent to a nursing home for people with mental impairment.

In Leiden 9 per cent of the elderly need domestic help; in Friesland the figure is 13 per cent. There is in this respect a big sex difference: in Leiden 5 per cent are aged men, but 12 per cent aged women; in Freisland the figure is 7 per cent and 18 per cent respectively for men and women; 80 per cent of this domestic help is given by family members.

Special housing for the aged (adapted or sheltered) is needed for at least 7 per cent of the age group 70–74; for 15 per cent of the age group of 75–79 and for 2 per cent of those over 80 years, apart from flats where some services are provided, i.e. cleaning and hot meals.

Survey of Health in Progressive Old Age (Beek and van Zonneveld 1976)

When the nationwide health interview and examination survey of 3149 old people by 374 general practitioners in 1955–1957 (van Zonneveld 1961) was complete, it was decided to re-examine the same population several times, involving the same general practitioners if possible for interviews and examinations and using the same questionnaire; often however, only a shorter questionnaire could be used.

Thus a longitudinal survey on health and psycho-social factors in the elderly was performed. The follow-up examinations took place after 5, 8, 11, 14, 16 and 17 years. Hence information was collected on *changes with age*, as well as discovering the *differences with age* using a cross-sectional study. The aim was to establish the relationship between the results obtained during the examinations (especially the first examination) and length of life (see Chapter 9).

Only a few of the more salient research results from the first four repeat examinations (in 11 years) will be given here.

Over the three follow-up phases the percentage of elderly people (65–75 years old) judged to be in good health by their own general practitioners at the first investigation had not decreased. This was not of course true for the older age groups.

Although feelings of loneliness and/or withdrawal were, as expected, unfavourably correlated with length of life, frequent contact with children appeared to be unimportant.

A drop in weight and height with age was noted; but no noticeable change was seen in haemoglobin levels, pulse rate, and systolic and diastolic blood pressure.

Over the past decade many of the general practitioners had considerably changed their ideas about the facilities they thought necessary for the elderly. This was partly because of increasing concern for the elderly and also because of service availability.

In the period 1960–1964 twice as many practitioners emphasized the need for more institutional facilities than emphasized the need for community facilities; in the period 1968–1972 these figures were the same. In the period 1960–1964 there was a greater demand for nursing homes than for residential homes: in the 1968–1972 period the reverse applied. There was also a demand for more facilities to enable admission of acutely handicapped elderly who lived independently.

CONCLUSION

These few examples should illustrate the use of the epidemiological measure of prevalence, particularly in relation to long-term conditions. The data from such prevalence studies provide information about the state of health and disease in a population at a particular time and about the health services required following such investigations. Often, however, surveys on incidence are necessary for a more detailed insight; for example, when changes in the processes of diseases, in type of treatment, and in attitudes take place in a relatively short period.

REFERENCES

Beek, A. & van Zonneveld, R. J. (1976) *De gezondheid in de voort-schrijdende ouderdom* (Health in progressive old age). Den Haag: Gezondheidsorganisatie TNO

Fennis, H. W. J. M. (1973) *Medische demografie van bejaarden. Bevolking, sterfte, ziekte en invaliditeit* (Medical demography of the aged. Population, mortality, morbidity and invalidity). Thesis Leiden. Leiden: Nederlands Instituut voor Praeventieve Geneeskunde TNO

Morris, G. V. (1975) *Uses of Epidemiology* (3rd Ed). Edinburgh: Churchill Livingstone

van Zonneveld, R. J. (1965/1966) *Langdurig zieken en hun behoeften* (Long-term patients and their needs). (Interim report 1: planning, procedure and follow-up of the survey). (2 vols) Leiden: Nederlands Instituut voor Praeventieve Geneeskunde TNO

van Zonneveld, R. J. (1961) *The Health of the Aged*; an investigation into the health and a number of social and psychological factors concerning 3 149 aged persons in the Netherlands, carried out by 374 general practitioners under the direction of the Organization for Health Research TNO. Assen: van Gorcum

van Zonneveld, R. J. (1954) *Gezondheidsproblemen bij bejaarden* (Health Problems of the Aged). Thesis Groningen. Assen: van Gorcum

SUGGESTED TEXTS FOR BACKGROUND READING

Alderson, M. (1976) *An Introduction to Epidemiology*. London: Macmillan Press

MacMahon, B. & Pugh, T. F. (1970) *Epidemiology: Principles and Methods*. Boston: Little Brown

Sturmans, F. (1975) *Epidemiologie en Medische Statistiek* (Epidemiology and Medical Statistics). Nijmegen: Dekker & Van de Vegt

van den Berg, J. W. H. & van Zonneveld, R. J. (1974) Epidemiologie. In *Sociale Geneeskunde* (Social Medicine) (4th Ed). van Zonneveld, R. J. (ed). Utrecht: Oosthoek, Scheltema & Holkema

SECTION 5

INCIDENCE STUDIES AND REGISTERS

CHAPTER 9

Incidence Studies

Alessandro Menotti

The incidence of a disease is a reasonable measure of its 'frequency'. It can be defined as the number of individuals becoming ill within a given period, taken as a proportion of those exposed to risk during that period. When the condition studied is chronic the denominator only includes individuals who have no clinical manifestations of the disease at entry.

Incidence can be measured by longitudinal studies on population samples or by continuous registration of the disease.

Accurate measurement of incidence relies on adequate sample size, appropriate follow-up, high participation and good measurement techniques. The measurement of incidence is useful for estimating the burden of disease in a population and it may also contribute to the search for causes through investigation of risk factors. Occasionally such measures are of immediate use in health care. The value of incidence measurements is limited by organizational and financial problems involved in conducting longitudinal studies.

DEFINITION OF INCIDENCE

Incidence is one of the most important measures of the frequency of a disease. It can be defined as the proportion of subjects who become ill within a certain period of time in relation to the total population at risk and can be expressed as:

$$\text{incidence} = \frac{\text{disease events}}{\text{population at risk}} \times 10^n \times \text{time period}$$

It is usually expressed per 100 or per 1000 (or other powers of 10) per year. For less common diseases the power of 10 is increased and the opposite applies for those that occur more often.

Incidence could be thought of as the 'production' of new cases of a disease by a population per unit of time. It is one of the variables which influence prevalence and it can be considered to be dynamic compared to prevalence which is a static measure.

THE FUNCTIONS OF INCIDENCE STUDIES

1. Incidence studies can be used to determine the number of cases occurring in a population over time. For some diseases this would provide a useful indicator of the burden of that disease on a community but such an indicator is often better provided by registration of the disease although this results in less accurate determination of the denominator i.e. the population at risk.

The indicators created in this way are particularly important in planning health services and particularly for preventive services. Chapters 10, 11 and 12 give further details.

2. They can be used to study disease occurrence in relation to different levels of 'risk factors' in individuals, subgroups or in entire populations. In this way possible causes of a particular disease can be sought: differences in incidence associated with different mean levels of a particular risk factor may suggest possible causal relationships, particularly if a given risk factor level is coupled with an extremely low incidence or when a risk factor level at the opposite extreme is associated with a high incidence.

3. They can be used to determine any trends in the occurrence or progress of a disease in relation to health services provided, preventive programmes and treatment given.

4. Studies of incidence can also provide a reference level of incidence for use in conducting controlled trials of population samples, for example, to determine the effectiveness of preventive measures.

CONDUCTING AN INCIDENCE STUDY

An incidence study is a longitudinal or prospective survey involving a number of steps which can be summarized as follows:

1. formulation of hypothesis (i.e. one of the four functions given above);
2. performance of a pilot study and the resulting analysis;
3. choice of a suitable population and a statistically valid sample;
4. recruitment of the population with preparation of a nominal list of those taking part:
5. definition of what is to be measured;

6. development of objective techniques, definition of conditions of measurement and of diagnostic criteria;

7. assessment of sensitivity, specificity, accuracy and precision of the methods, training of personnel and testing of methods;

8. primary examination of the selected population;

9. determination of response rates;

10. follow-up of non-respondents;

11. further examinations;

12. final examination;

13. analysis and interpretation.

Most of these steps have methodological problems which are described elsewhere in this book. Problems connected with the choice of the population, the sample size and others will be dealt with here.

Some aspects of incidence require special attention. These include the source of the study, the follow-up system and the mechanism for eliciting new cases of a disease.

SOURCE OF THE STUDY AND CHARACTERISTICS OF THE DENOMINATOR

A major feature of incidence studies is that there must be sufficient individuals in a study to obtain adequate numbers who develop the disease or condition in question within the study period. Several different population groups may be used for study purposes. They may be: whole communities; occupational groups; medical care groups; people insured privately or by social security schemes; and self-selected or other special groups.

Whole communities have the advantage of being the most representative; either the entire community can be examined or samples can be drawn (i.e. chunk sample) after definition of a geographical and/or administrative base (Keys et al 1966). Their disadvantage is that participation might be low, particularly if the sample is drawn from a large city.

Occupational groups are easy to recruit, individuals are often more willing to participate and there may be built-in information systems to enable easy follow-up. However occupational groups may have special problems and characteristics which do not exist in the general population. Examples of incidence studies in occupational groups include local and international surveys. A famous local study of the incidence of coronary heart disease among bus drivers and conductors in London was performed by Morris et al (1966). International comparisons have been made between, for example, United States and Italian railroad workers within the 'Seven Countries Study' (Keys 1970).

People enrolled in prepaid medical care, for example in general practice, have the advantage of being easy to contact initially through the general practitioner and easy to follow up through the practice registration system. The Royal College of General Practitioners in the United Kingdom undertook a national morbidity survey by collecting records of consultations taking place in over 100 practices in a year (OPCS 1974). Similar studies can be applied to members of private life insurance or compulsory social security schemes.

Special and self-selected groups tend to be rather unrepresentative of a general population, but good studies have been conducted in this type of sample, for example among blood donors (Oliver 1970) or those undergoing voluntary screenings for cancer (Rinzler 1968). It should be possible to identify differences in characteristics compared with the general population.

Since the denominator of incidence is defined as the population at risk of developing the 'event' as given by the numerator, all individuals in the denominator must have equal potential for entering the disease or 'event' status as defined for the study purpose.

The structure of the denominator depends on the purpose of the survey. A study with a scientific purpose, such as measuring and comparing the amount of disease occurring in different population groups, or determining the role of supposed risk factors, must exclude subjects who already have the disease at entry to the study, particularly if a chronic disease is being studied. In this case the population will be described as disease-free; this selection must be done at the initial examination.

In other studies, like those simply based on registration, there is no way of excluding the current cases of disease: if the study involves special population groups, insured groups or people at special risk, previous medical records may define these cases, even without an entry examination in the study.

FOLLOW-UP AND THE CHARACTERISTICS OF THE NUMERATOR

Whether the sample has been drawn from the general population or consists of a special group, the follow-up is aimed at determining the outcome for each individual, as shown by appearance of the disease or death. The completeness of such ascertainment for individuals should not be affected by membership or non-membership of particular subgroups of the population.

In some cases outcome can be elicited from routine procedures independent of the fact that the subjects are part of a special study. Such procedures would include:

death records;
hospital records;
registered diseases;
general practitioner records;
diseases reported to health authorities;
reports of absenteeism from work or school;
and medical statistics of health services.

By using these routine sources it is sometimes possible to perform a retrospective longitudinal study by reconstructing both the numerator and the denominator of incidence from past medical records. This is only suitable for answering some specific questions and care should be taken in the validation of such studies. An example is the study of former students at Harvard University who were classified as athletes or non-athletes. The outcome for these two groups could be described in terms of the incidence of cardiovascular disease and general mortality (Pedelnak 1972).

In general all these sources of information of event data lack completeness and accuracy. To be efficient a routine source of information must reveal the majority of cases or deaths which occur in the particular cohort. Where there has been a change of occupation, emigration from the study area, or incomplete reporting this may not occur.

A precise and sophisticated way of collecting data is by periodic examinations of all members of the sample using the same procedure as at entry examination. This is obviously expensive and has the disadvantage of a decreasing response rate over time with increasing self-selection among responders. However in well-conducted studies this is the ideal method of data collection. After the respondents have been examined, every effort should be made to collect, by direct or indirect means, maximum information from non-respondents. Personal contacts, home visits, letters to the individuals, to the family, to the register office and contacts with any possible witness and source of information, may all be used with the overall aim of obtaining 100 per cent participation at follow-up. Table 1 gives an example of a good response rate after special efforts have been made. It shows the response to a 10-year follow-up

Table 1. *Example of participation rate in a 10-year follow-up examination in a study of cardiovascular disease incidence in two rural population groups in Italy (Source: Menotti and Puddu 1973)*

Examined at entry	1717 (98.7% of sample)
Deaths ascertained with full information about cause	211
Survivors	1506
Emigrants from area	226 (15% of survivors)
Respondents to 10-year examination (including some emigrants)	1408 (93.5% of survivors)
Non-respondents	98 (6.5% of survivors)
Information obtained by letter about non-respondents	54 (55.1% of non-respondents)
Indirect information about non-respondents	13 (13.3% of non-respondents)
No information except about status of non-respondents	31 (31.6% of non-respondents)

examination of 1717 men from demographic samples of rural areas of Northern and Central Italy, within an incidence study of cardiovascular disease (Menotti and Puddu 1973).

In general a study which aims at determining incidence for comparative purposes, or at identification of risk factors, should collect only clean cases, that is individuals who develop the disease in question for the first time. This particularly applies to chronic conditions. Surveys intended to provide information about the burden of the disease on the community or to help in the planning of health services, must take into account all disease events such as relapses or recurrences. The technique for counting cases occurring over time to provide the numerator varies according to the disease in question. Some acute diseases like the common cold, influenza, minor accidents, or even serious infectious illnesses of short duration which leave no indication that the condition has occurred can only be assessed by frequent or even continuous monitoring of every individual. Alternatively information could be given by health personnel or simply recalled on questionnaires at a later date. In the latter situation diagnosis becomes less certain, unless specific changes of a biochemical or immunological nature in the blood, or visible scars and other signs remain to allow recognition of the healed disease or to confirm the reported history.

Usually a chronic disease which starts with a clinically overt period is easily recognized even when checks on the individuals at risk are infrequent, but exact timing of disease initiation may be difficult. Cases of chronic bronchitis, or of gastric ulcer are good examples. Some chronic diseases may over time lose the objective evidence of their existence and hence recognition may become more difficult, for example if field examinations are performed after a long period. As a result diagnosis following field examination becomes 'softer' and less certain. An example of this is minor myocardial infarction for which electro-cardiographic evidence may disappear after a time, and only reported history or hospital documentation for the actual event will be available. There is no doubt however that chronic coronary heart disease still exists, although 'recovery' is apparently complete.

Another relevant problem in incidence studies of myocardial infarction and also of cerebrovascular accidents, some serious traumas and poisonings is that a new case can become a death within a shorter period than the time lapse for any periodic or systematic direct check of the population at risk. For example it is well documented that 25 per cent or more of heart attack cases die within two hours of the onset of symptoms and many more die within 24 hours of onset. Much the same applies to cerebrovascular accidents and, to a lesser extent to road accidents, poisoning, and other violent causes. It is quite clear however that such cases belong to the incidence numerator and therefore particular care must be taken to ensure their detection outside the normal periodical check of surviving members of a population.

TIME LAPSE, INCIDENCE SIZE AND STUDY POPULATION SIZE

Incidence is normally expressed per 10^n per year: usually an incidence study is conducted for periods of at least a year. The minimum duration of a study depends on two variables—the expected incidence and the size of the population at risk: duration must be inversely proportional to both. In general for common conditions or for large populations at risk, a duration of one year is sufficient (e.g. for common cold in a sizeable population; or myocardial infarction in an adult population of 10 000 or even 100 000). For rare conditions or small samples the duration of the study must be longer and the population must be followed for several years in order to find enough cases for analysis and comparison.

It must be remembered that the majority of diseases which represent common epidemiological problems are uncommon with the exception of conditions like sore throat, the common cold, acute bronchitis, infections of the upper respiratory tract, dental caries, and minor accidents. For example the incidence of myocardial infarction in the most vulnerable populations throughout the world—that is the middle-aged—is roughly one per cent per year (Keys 1970). But to obtain 50 cases of leukaemia within one year would require a population of almost a million people. This shows how large samples or long study periods are needed to collect adequate case numbers (MacMahon 1960). This must be remembered when planning a study in relation to choice of the sample, its size and duration.

INCIDENCE IN NON-RESPONDENTS

Problems may arise if follow-up is incomplete, because a valid estimate of incidence is needed and it is reasonable to suspect that non-respondents have a different incidence of disease: if a rare condition is being studied loss of even a single case presents a major problem. There are several ways of tackling the situation. If the incidence rate includes in the denominator all men enrolled including those lost to follow-up, an estimate of minimum incidence can be obtained. If the denominator only includes individuals with complete follow-up it is automatically assumed that incidence rate in non-respondents is equal to that of respondents. When a study is spread over several years and, events are registered by each year, if follow-up has not been possible a certain drop-out rate must be accepted. In this case incidence is given as persons per year of exposure and the denominator takes into account the annual weighted mean duration of exposure to risk of the study population.

It is possible but unlikely that all subjects lost to follow-up have developed the disease, in which case the rate given would be the so-called 'maximum incidence'.

However rather than using maximum or minimum incidence it may be more reasonable to consider an alternative hypothesis. For example, it might be assumed that non-respondents have an incidence rate double or half that of respondents. An example is given in Table 2. In general when the overall incidence rate is low and follow-up occurs for a fairly large proportion of the population, overestimation is less of a problem than underestimation. However, good studies can be carried out even if substantial losses to follow-up occur. A good example is the Framingham study of coronary heart disease, where only 68.6 per cent of the chosen population was examined at entry to the study (Rose and Blackburn 1968).

Table 2. *Theoretical hypothesis of incidence rate with non-respondents at follow-up (Based on a group of 1200 individuals with 1000 respondents, 200 non-respondents and 50 observed cases)*

Observed incidence	50/1000 = 0.050
Minimum incidence	50/1200 = 0.042
Maximum incidence	250/1200 = 0.208
True incidence	10 + 50/1200 = 0.050
non-respondents have *the same*	(observed incidence estimate
incidence as respondents	is correct)
True incidence	20 + 50/1200 = 0.058
non-respondents have *double*	(observed incidence underestimates
the incidence of respondents	true incidence by 8%)
True incidence	5 + 50/1200 = 0.048
non-respondents have *half*	(observed incidence overestimates
the incidence of respondents	true incidence by 2%)

THE SEARCH FOR RISK FACTORS

One of the main functions of incidence studies is identification of risk factors, that is the measurable characteristics at an individual or collective level which, in individuals or populations without clinical manifestations of the disease, enable detection of those individuals or subgroups who have a higher risk of developing the disease within a certain period of time; or identification of the population groups in which the disease in question will be more common in the near future, because of the presence of these risk factors in that population. For most morbid conditions multifactorial prediction of disease occurrence is the most appropriate approach.

Briefly, the principles and procedures for the identification of risk factors can be described as follows:

On the basis of a hypothesis drawn from clinical experience, from health statistics or previous research, certain individual characteristics are suspected to be risk factors. A longitudinal study is set up and at entry examination, measurements of the suspect risk factors are obtained; the individuals who already have the disease under investigation are excluded. After an appropriate follow-up period the incidence data will be analysed as a function of different levels of the risk factor (or in the case of a discrete dichotomic characteristic as a function of its presence or absence). For factors with a continuous distribution a number of arbitrary classes can be defined and the number of individuals examined at entry will represent, for each class, the denominator of a rate whose numerator is given by the number of cases occurring in that class. The rate will be the incidence of the disease or the risk of developing it for

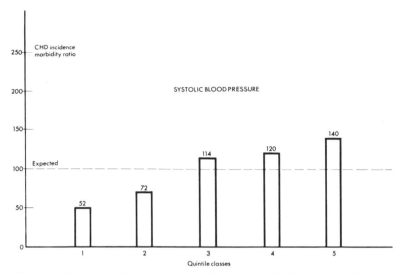

Figure 1. Example of the relationship between a risk factor (systolic blood pressure) and the incidence of coronary heart disease in subgroups of subjects with different levels of the risk factor belonging to the same population group. The Seven Countries Study, Italian rural areas, five-year follow-up (Source: Keys 1970)

each level of the risk factor. Quantile classes of the risk factor (denominator) may make the analysis easier since in this case the numerator alone indicates the presence or absence of a disease trend with increasing or decreasing levels of the factor in question (Figure 1).

Obviously the null hypothesis is that no difference in incidence will be found in different classes of the risk factor distribution. This *unconditional* risk or probability is given by the overall incidence rate for all the observations; the *conditional* risk for each class is given by the rate as computed above; whereas the *relative* risk is given by the ratio between two levels of conditional risk (or between any level and the unconditional risk).

Tests to compare the rates for extreme classes of the distribution or to analyse the overall trend may elicit statistically significant differences in risk between different levels of risk factors.

Sometimes when whole population samples or groups are compared instead of subgroups of a single population, the relationship between factors and risk is found by plotting the mean or median levels of the factors against the incidence rate for each population group (Figure 2).

Schematically there might be several types of relationship between

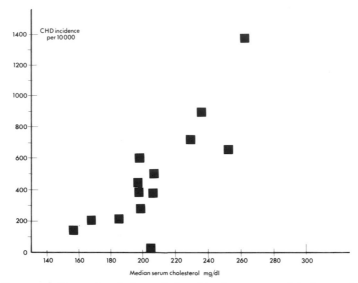

Figure 2. Example of the relationship between a risk factor (serum cholesterol) and the incidence of coronary heart disease in 14 different population groups, represented by their median levels of the risk factor and their overall incidence. The Seven Countries Study, five-year follow-up (Modified from Keys 1970 and reproduced with permission from the American Heart Association Inc., Dallas, Texas)

factors and disease. They may be positive or negative, and within each class they can be expressed mathematically by a straight line, by an exponential or parabolic curve or by other more complex equations.

The above description of risk-factor identification illustrates the process of univariate analysis which considers only one factor at a time and does not allow for the presence of others.

'Multivariate analysis' of incidence as a function of risk factors might be preceded by standardization of incidence rates examined as a function of one factor by the distribution of another. A further similar step involves analysis of cross-classifications which soon becomes impossible as the number of factors and the number of classes for each factor increase. A large number of cases and a large sample are required to fill up all the possible cells in the cross-classification.

Proper multivariate analysis is based on mathematical models which enable estimation of the disease (incidence or risk) as a function of several factors at the same time. For each factor a coefficient is found

Table 3. *Example of a multiple logistic solution for the estimation of coronary risk* (the 'Seven Countries Study' European cohorts of men aged 40–59 at entry, followed for five years). Prediction of incidence cases of 'any-criteria coronary heart disease' in men CHD-free at entry. Population at risk = 8728; cases = 405 (*Source: Keys et al 1972*)

Risk factors	Coefficients	p of t value
Age in years	0.066	0.001
Systolic blood pressure mm Hg	0.019	0.001
Serum cholesterol mg/dl	0.008	0.001
Smoking habits (score)	0.031	0.05
Body mass index (weight in kg/height in m)	0.026	n.s.
Constant	−11.888	—

Distribution of observed cases in decile classes of estimated risk obtained by applying the coefficients to the same population	Decile	Cases
	1	9
	2	19
	3	16
	4	22
	5	27
	6	37
	7	34
	8	53
	9	78
	10	110

indicating the relative weight or contribution to risk, with all other factors kept equal. Discrimination of cases from non-cases can be attempted by applying the coefficients back to the same or to other populations and, although imperfect, it might be impressive when it is possible to collect as many cases as possible in the extreme right of the distribution of the estimated risk.

The most exploited models are:

the linear multiple regression $y = a + \Sigma b_i x_i$;

the corresponding discriminant function $y = z + \Sigma x_i b_i$;

and the multiple logistic function $y = [1 + \exp-(a + \Sigma b_i x_i)]^{-1}$.

The advantage of the last is it expresses the disease in terms of probabilities.

An example of the solution of a multiple logistic function for the estimation of coronary risk is given in Table 3. The relative 'weight' of single factors for predicting the disease (that is discriminating cases from non-cases) is given by the coefficients and by the p of their t value; the distribution of observed cases of decile classes of estimated risk are illustrated as well showing that relative risk between extreme classes is fairly substantial.

Such models require special care and attention in the interpretation of their results to be put to satisfactory use. Further details about their use can be found in the following publications: Truett, Cornfield and Kannel 1967; Walker and Duncan 1967; Keys et al 1972.

The causative role of risk factors cannot be fully demonstrated by incidence studies despite the fact that they provide some suggestive evidence; their main role is that of a tool for accurate prediction of the disease and for selection of high risk individuals or populations with regard to preventive treatment. The final proof of causation is only obtained from experimental studies of primary prevention which are described in Section 7 on causation and control.

PROBLEMS CONNECTED WITH INCIDENCE STUDIES AND IMPLICATIONS FOR HEALTH CARE

Studies of incidence have the main advantage of providing a comprehensive measure of the frequency of a disease and the basis for the evaluation of characteristics thought to be risk factors on an individual or a population basis. Both types of evaluation are important for explanation of a causative hypothesis. In addition they avoid the problems connected with the interpretation of prevalence, as a measure of frequency of disease, and of the relationships between suspected risk factors and prevalence cases which are often equivocal and misleading. This is mainly so when dealing with diseases characterized by high early fatality, and also when risk factor levels vary to produce differing severity of the disease or even change after the occurrence of the disease as a result of biological and/or iatrogenic aspects.

Because of their long duration, complexity and high cost, incidence studies of the cohort type mainly serve to answer specific scientific questions in the field of causation and prevention of diseases, only rarely can they be implemented in the field of health care.

However there are several examples in the literature where relatively short term surveys have provided valuable information for immediate use in general health care. An example is the study by Bennett et al (1968) of the care of the elderly in residential homes. It was shown that incidence of hip fractures was higher in residents of old people's homes than in the general population of the same age and sex. A clear need for better assistance in such homes emerged from the study.

Incidence studies also have several disadvantages. They are usually of long duration, and may even last for quinquennia or decades; the organization of long term follow-up is often difficult and cumbersome; there is a strong likelihood that people will be unable to answer the questions asked and answers may be collected only after many years of effort; there is also the possibility of losing a sizeable proportion of at-risk individuals at long-term follow-up which would reduce the strength of the statistical analysis; also the financial input is often enormous and sometimes prohibitive.

Before embarking on a longitudinal study the advantages and disadvantages must be weighed against the value of the question for which an answer is sought and the likelihood of the answer being definitive—that is either positive or negative.

REFERENCES

Bennett, A. E., Deane, M., Elliot, A. & Holland, W. W. (1968) Care of old people in residential homes. *British Journal of Preventive & Social Medicine*, *22*, 193

Keys, A., Aravanis, C., Blackburn, H. W., van Buchem, F. S. P., Buzina, R., Djordjevic, B. S., Dontas, A. S., Fidanza, F., Karvonen, M. J., Kimura, N., Lekos, D., Monti, M., Puddu, V. & Taylor, H. L. (1966) Epidemiological studies related to coronary heart disease: Characteristics of men aged 40–59 in Seven Countries. *Acta Medica Scandinavica*, *181*, Supplement 460

Keys, A., Aravanis, C., Blackburn, H., van Buchem, F. S. P., Buzina, R., Djordjevic, B. S. , Fidanza, F., Karvonen, M., Menotti, A., Puddu, V. & Taylor, H. (1972) The probability of middle-aged men developing coronary heart disease in five years. *Circulation*, *45*, 815

Keys, A. (ed) (1970) Coronary heart disease in seven countries. *Circulation*, *41*, Supplement 1

MacMahon, B., Pugh, T. F. & Ipsen, J. (1960) *Epidemiologic Methods.* London: Churchill

Menotti, A. & Puddu, V. (1973) Epidemiology of coronary heart disease. A 10 year study in two Italian rural population groups. *Acta Cardiologica*, *28*, 66

Morris, J. N., Kagan, A., Pattison, D. C., Gardner, M. J. & Raffle, P. A. B. (1966) Incidence and prediction of ischaemic heart disease in London busmen. *Lancet*, *2*, 553

Oliver, M. F. (1970) A primary prevention trial using clofibrate to lower hyperlipidemia. In *Atherosclerosis:* Proceedings of the Second International Symposium. Jones, M. F. (ed). New York: Springer-Verlag, p. 582

OPCS (1974) *Morbidity Statistics from General Practice. Second National Study 1970–71.* Studies on Medical and Population Subjects No. 26. London: HMSO

Pedelnak, A. P. (1972) Longevity and cardiovascular mortality among former college athletes. *Circulation*, *46*, 649

Rinzler, S. H. (1968) Primary prevention of coronary heart disease by diet. *Bulletin of New York Academy of Medicine*, *44*, 936

Truett, J., Cornfield, J. & Kannel, W. (1967) A multivariate analysis of the risk of coronary heart disease in Framingham. *Journal of Chronic Diseases*, *20*, 511

Walker, S. H. & Duncan, D. B. (1967) Estimation of the probability of an event as a function of several independent variables. *Biometrika*, *54*, 167

WHO (1976) *Myocardial Infarction Community Registers*. Public Health in Europe 5. Copenhagen: World Health Organization, Regional Office for Europe

SUGGESTED TEXTS FOR BACKGROUND READING

Abramson, J. H. (1974) *Survey Methods in Community Medicine*. Edinburgh: Churchill Livingstone

Barker, D. J. P. & Rose, G. (1976) *Epidemiology in Medical Practice*. Edinburgh: Churchill Livingstone

MacMahon, B. & Pugh, T. F. (1970) *Epidemiology: principles and methods*. Boston: Little Brown

Morris, J. N. (1975) *Uses of Epidemiology*. Edinburgh: Churchill Livingstone

Rose, G. A. & Blackburn, H. (1968) *Cardiovascular Survey Methods*. Geneva: World Health Organization

WHO (1967) Epidemiological Methods in the Study of Chronic Diseases. *World Health Organization Technical Report Series*, No. 365

Introduction to Registers

The answer to the question, why should three chapters on registers be included in a section on incidence studies, is simply that in certain instances a register is the most successful method for establishing the incidence of a condition. Doll (1972) in a discussion on sources of data on cancer concludes that incidence rates obtained from routine cancer registration or by a special research project run for a limited period in a defined area, are probably the data of choice and correspond very closely to the true incidence of the disease. This applies to conditions other than cancer, for example tuberculosis, ischaemic heart disease and strokes.

The principal objectives of registers can be summarized as collating information collected from defined groups over time, which may be used in the prevention or treatment of disease, the provision of after care, the monitoring of changing patterns of disease and medical care, and the evaluation and planning of services. The most successful registers seem to be those in which the data collected are accurate, restricted to the essentials, and meet a need that cannot be satisfied in any other way. Those set up to study changing patterns of disease and the possible aetiological factors leading to these changes must be based on defined populations and be as complete as possible. To achieve this, information must be collected from as many sources as possible and checked for completeness and duplication. The three registers discussed in this section, the Danish Tuberculosis Index, the Danish Cancer Register and the WHO Ischaemic Heart Disease Register are examples of registers that successfully meet these objectives. Other registers have been set up but have failed; many of these have attempted to meet rather ill-defined needs, such as the provision of educational tools and the advancement of teaching and research.

Registers cover a variety of interests, for example, in preventive medicine, for the organization and delivery of immunization and screening programmes. Disease-specific registers include those for blindness, psychiatric disorders, ischaemic heart disease, stroke, cancer and tuberculosis, and they were among the earliest to be set up: they are used both in aetiological studies and in the planning and delivery of care.

Treatment registers provide a continuing list and follow-up of all individuals with certain categories of disease in a defined setting; they are intended to provide information likely to be useful in clinical practice. After care registers may simply act as information centres or may be part of the machinery of giving after care, such as the Register of Disabled Persons in which registration is voluntary, but those on the register may go to Industrial Rehabilitation Units and be employed under special provisions.

There is a great variety of at-risk registers which work with varying degrees of success: for example, children at risk of abuse, or neglect; certain workers at risk from occupational hazards; and people at risk for medical reasons, e.g. diabetics, those on steroid treatment, and those with drug hypersensitivity. This last at-risk register, 'Medic-Alert', is one of the largest and most active of all registers.

Some long-term prospective studies have been based on registers, for example the Thousand Families Study (Spence et al 1964) and the National Child Development Study (Davie, Butler and Goldstein 1972).

Registers of specific information generally have two objectives: to establish the prevalence of a condition; and to act as information centres. They have met with varying degrees of success, which often depends on the urgency of the need for the information.

REFERENCES

Davie, R., Butler, N. & Goldstein, H. (1972) *From Birth to Seven*. London: Longman

Doll, R. (1972) Cancer in five continents. *Proceedings of the Royal Society of Medicine*, 65, 49

Spence, J., Walton, W. S., Miller, F. J. W. & Court, S. D. M. (1964) *A Thousand Families in Newcastle upon Tyne*. London: Oxford University Press

Epidemiological Parameters for the Public Health Evaluation of a Chronic Disease[1]

Ole Horwitz

In 1921 a national register of tuberculosis in Denmark was established to record all cases of active tuberculosis. The organization and management of the register has been changed over the years in order to maximize the information produced, and minimize the expenditure and time lag between reporting and production of statistics. A model has been developed on the basis of this material showing the dynamic interplay between disease, cure and death. It describes the indices which are of immediate public health significance; the infection rate, incidence and prevalence, the cure rate and excess mortality among sick patients, and the relapse rate and excess mortality among patients with arrested disease. The different indices can be used to determine priorities within the medical services; to identify high-risk groups in need of surveillance; and to assess the existing medical programme.

INTRODUCTION

According to the classic literature, the tuberculosis problem was visualized as a lake, with an inflow of sick patients and an outflow of cured and dead cases; the water level rose and fell with the shifting volumes of inflow and outflow. With the establishment of the centralized Danish reporting system for tuberculosis it became possible to show this dynamic interplay between disease, cure and death, and to illustrate—in numerical terms—parameters describing the epidemiology of the disease and its natural course. Moreover, this registration system provided the health administrator with data assessing treatment regimens and the clinician

[1] This is an updated and revised version of the article originally published in *American Journal of Epidemiology* (1973) 97, 148

with some of the data needed for projecting a prognosis for his individual patients.

THE REGISTRATION SYSTEM

Since the turn of the century, it has been compulsory in Denmark to report active cases of pulmonary tuberculosis. The notifications collected from the doctors and hospitals were kept in local files. This material did not allow a reliable estimate of the diseases as a nationwide problem, since the same patient might be reported several times in different locations; to remedy this, a central register was established in 1921, covering the entire country. There was a continuous and large inflow of notifications into the register, whereas notifications were only removed in case of death from tuberculosis; the register therefore grew constantly. In the 1930s, a new administrative regulation allowed for notifications to be removed after they had been filed for more than eight years. The number of cards in the register then gave a better estimate of the total number of persons who suffered from the disease, but it did not give correct information about the individual patient: some who were listed were in fact cured or had died from other diseases; conversely, some who had been removed were still sick with active disease.

By the end of the 1940s there were chest clinics throughout Denmark. Almost all tuberculosis patients were treated and controlled by the clinics and so fairly complete data became available. It was therefore agreed to give up the old book-keeping system on the central file. Instead, chest physicians were asked to report what happened to the patients, in terms of arrest of the disease or death, after they had been first reported to the register. From 1950 to 1972, the criterion for cure was that tubercle bacilli were not demonstrated over the three consecutive years after cessation of treatment. In 1972 a new criterion for cure was adopted, namely discontinuance of treatment. The disease was now classified as 'active' as long as the patient was under a drug regimen; the disease was registered as 'cured' when treatment stopped. In order to secure reliable data, the treatment status of each patient is centrally recorded each year by means of a nationwide surveillance system, established and conducted by the Danish Institute for Clinical Epidemiology.

INFECTION RATE

This rate measures how often individuals in the general population are infected with tubercle bacilli; it is generally expressed as the number of new tuberculin reactors recorded in one year among 1000 negative individuals. The infection rate is often considered a reliable index of the tuberculosis problem, but this is so with strong modifications. Cross-sensitivity to atypical mycobacteria presents a problem in identifying true infection with human tubercle bacilli in the subtropical areas; infection through milk with bovine bacilli poses the same problem, and so does the widespread use of BCG vaccination. The risk of developing pulmonary tuberculosis by those sensitized to atypical or bovine myco-bacteria is almost nil; hence, the total number of tuberculin reactors does not provide a valid estimate of the past, the present or the future tubercle problem. In addition studies from the few countries with valid data have shown that morbidity and infection rates do not necessarily vary in parallel. Thus, the incidence and mortality of tuberculosis increased in Holland during wartime, whereas the infection rate continued to drop (Styblo, Meijer and Sutherland 1969); in Greenland, where the infection is due only to human tubercle bacillus, the incidence among tuberculin reactors was many times higher than in Denmark, even in groups with the same roentgenological findings (Horwitz 1972).

Spot checks in Danish districts where BCG is administered only to school-leavers have provided an estimate of the infection rate among young children—in the order of 1 per 5000 or even lower. This low infection rate in young children suggests that the tuberculosis problem in Denmark is almost solved. Morbidity and mortality data, as shown below, give a different picture—the disease is still a public health problem.

INCIDENCE

Figure 1 illustrates the present tubercle situation in Denmark with a total population of five million. The figure depicts the tuberculosis problem as a series of pools representing different population groups, and a series of flows representing those whose health changed during the year. The flow of sick patients arising in the general population, 'first timers', represents those who developed active tuberculosis for the first time; the stream of cases which flows from the Pool of Previous Cases, represents the relapses. The input of 540 cases represents the incidence; it is made up of 460 first timers and 80 relapses, corresponding to a rate of 11 per 100000. In many countries the official statistics include only the first-time cases, but relapses are just as infectious and need just as much care and control as the first timers. It is therefore most realistic and meaningful to use the combined rate of new plus reactivated cases as the indication for 'incidence'.

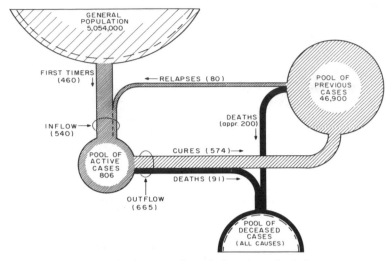

Figure 1. The flows and pools in tuberculosis in 1975

PREVALENCE

Whereas the number of new cases is a sensitive indicator of the morbidity for acute conditions such as measles, it is not sufficient for chronic diseases. Here, long-term cases pose a great part of the problem. Two slightly different indices gauge this rate: the 'point-prevalence' which is based on a count of all patients on a given day, and the 'period-prevalence' which indicates how many people suffered from the disease during a year. Figure 1 shows that on 1 January 1975, a total of 806 cases were listed in the Pool of Active Cases, corresponding to a point-prevalence of 16 per 100000. The period-prevalence was 27 per 100000: this rate is based on the 806 patients who were in the Pool of Active Cases at the beginning of 1975 plus the 540 patients who entered it during that year.

MORTALITY AND LETHALITY

During 1975 a total of 91 patients died; this figure includes patients in whom pulmonary tuberculosis was the primary cause of death as well as those where it was only a contributory cause. From among the 91 deaths, the doctors had stated on the death certificate that 37 cases died *from* tuberculosis which gives a mortality rate of 0.7 per 100000. The remaining 54 patients died *with* tuberculosis. In some cases it may be simple to decide the cause of death, e.g. when tuberculosis is the only manifest disease at the time of death. The decision becomes more

Table 1. *Excess mortality for patients of all ages with active tuberculosis in Denmark (1975)*

Deaths (n)	Observed	91
	Expected	21
Excess	Difference[a]	70
	Ratio[b]	4.3

[a] Observed number − expected number
[b] Observed number ÷ expected number

difficult, or even impossible, when competing potentially lethal diseases coexist. Other factors, such as the central coding of the death certificate, may further change the cause of death given by the physician: 'senility', for instance, is not accepted as the main cause of death, if other diseases are mentioned on the certificate. As a result mortality data may be more fragile than is generally considered.

The classic measure of the severity of a disease is the lethality, which indicates how many patients die from it. For chronic diseases, the period over which patients are observed must be specified—one year has been selected for this analysis. During 1975, a total of 37 deaths from tuberculosis were reported; these deaths occurred among the 1346 patients who were in the Incidence Stream and the Pool of Active Cases; this gives a lethality of 2.7 per cent. Whether this should be judged as high or low depends upon the number of deaths which normally would have occurred; the 'excess mortality' may be used to gauge the difference more clearly. The observed number of deaths, 91, shown in Table 1 refers to the deaths in 1975 from all causes among all the patients with active tuberculosis in any age group. The expected number of deaths was 21. (This number was found by dividing the patients in the Incidence Stream and the Pool of Active Cases by sex and age and applying the sex/age-specific death rates from all causes in the general population on each group; summing over all the cells gives the total number of expected deaths.) The excess might be measured as the difference between the observed and expected number which was 70. The excess might also be estimated from the ratio between observed and expected deaths which was 4.3. In other words, mortality among tuberculosis patients is many times higher than in a corresponding group of normal people. The implications of the excess is further evaluated in Figure 2 which shows the age distribution of observed and expected deaths. Although the highest rates are in the elderly, quite a number of deaths occurred in middle age. The number of years which the 70 'excess deaths' normally would have lived have

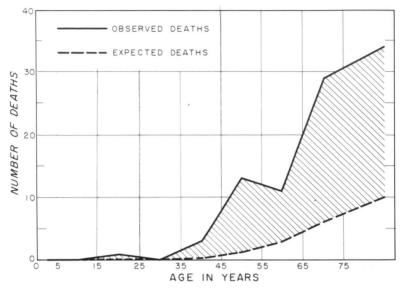

Figure 2. The observed and expected number of deaths among tuber-culosis patients, by age, Denmark 1975

been calculated from the official tables on life expectancy; taken alto-gether, they would have lived 1045 years. This means that the longevity for the 1346 tubercle patients in the Incidence Stream and the Pool of Active Cases, was shortened by nine months on average. If the 1045 lost years are related to the total sum of years which the 1346 infected patients would have experienced if they had not had tuberculosis, their life expectancy would be diminished by 3.4 per cent.

PROGNOSIS

One of the most important tasks for the clinician, as well as the public health administrator, is to project a prognosis. But what is actually meant by this term, and how do we measure it? Some of the indices which seem most useful are presented in the following: attack rate among infected individuals; cure and death rates for patients; the relapse rate among cured patients and their excess mortality.

Attack rate among infected individuals. The implication of being in-fected with tubercle bacilli should be evaluated by a lifelong follow-up of a representative group of recently infected individuals. The material from the Danish mass screening programme of 1950–1952 may shed some light

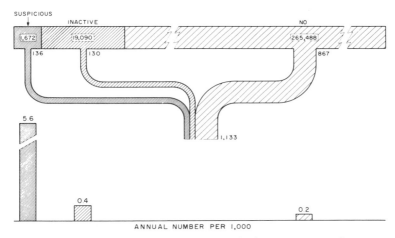

Figure 3. Incidence of pulmonary tuberculosis among natural reactors according to x-ray findings at mass campaign; 16 years of follow-up

on this problem. Among the attenders, a total of 286 250 natural reactors were identified in the 15–44 year age group; none of them had ever had tuberculosis and none of them were vaccinated with BCG. In the next 16 years a total of 1133 cases of tuberculosis were diagnosed in the study population, giving an annual risk of 0.3 per 1000. This rate is too low to require public health action, such as routine examination or chemo-prophylaxis. Figure 3 shows that the risk varied considerably according to initial chest x-ray findings: those with suspicious x-ray lesions at the time of a mass campaign had the highest annual rate (5.6 per 1000); and those with a normal chest roentgenogram had the lowest rate (0.2 per 1000). It would seem reasonable to maintain close surveillance in the former group, but not in the latter.

Cure and death rates. Figure 1 showed that 574 patients were cured and 91 died among all the patients with active tuberculosis. This cor-responds to a crude cure rate of 43 per cent and a crude death rate of 7 per cent. This data can be made much more informative by using a decrement table, as illustrated for a hypothetical group of patients in Table 2. The patients are grouped according to duration of disease: 810 cases were newly diagnosed; 623 had been sick for one year; 411 for two years, etc. The number of deaths occurring during the year of observation is given in column 3. The mortality in each group is then computed from the numbers in columns 2 and 3. Let us now assume that we had a cohort of 1000 new cases. When are they likely to die? During the first year the

Table 2. *Hypothetical survival table*

Duration (years)	Observed			Expected	
	No. of patients at onset of year	No. of deaths	Mortality (%)	No. of patients at onset of year	No. of deaths
1	810	130	16	1000	160
2	623	62	10	840	84
3	411	23	5	756	38
4	265	16	6	718	43

mortality rate was 16 per cent; hence 160 will die and 840 remain alive. Applying the death rate for the second year, 10 per cent, to this group gives 84 deaths, leaving 756 individuals. The computations are continued in this way until all 1000 patients are dead.

Similarly, patients in the Pool of Active Cases were divided by duration of diseases into cases on file for one year, two years, etc. Cure and death rates in each group were then computed from the information received through the reporting system. The observed rates were combined in a decrement table in which the patients were candidates not only for death but also for cure. Figure 4 shows the forecast for 100 newly reported cases: 3½ years after the report 16 per cent had died, 81 per cent were cured, and 3 per cent were chronically sick. Figure 4 shows the average for all patients but it varies by age and severity of disease: for example, the cure rate in middle-aged patients with minimal disease was twice the rate for those with advanced disease; conversely, their mortality rate was one-third of that for those with advanced disease. This finding is hardly surprising, but the method has the advantage of measuring in quantitative terms how great the actual differences are.

Relapse rate and excess mortality among cured patients. Among the 46900 cases who were in the Pool of Previous Cases on 1 January 1975, a total of 80 suffered a relapse during the year. The incidence among the previous cases is thus 1.7 per 1000, or 19 times higher than the rate in the general population. A special analysis of the mortality from all causes among cured patients showed that the rate was 34 per cent higher than expected, the expected rate being the mortality in a group of normal persons with the same sex and age set-up as the patients. The excess incidence and the excess mortality among cured patients can be considered as the ultimate toll of tubercle bacillus.

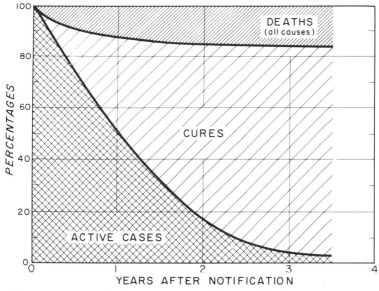

Figure 4. Prognosis for new cases (all ages) of pulmonary tuberculosis

DISCUSSION

The ever-increasing demands for public services of all kinds, be it transportation, housing, social welfare, or education, have limited the resources available for the medical system. It is now imperative for planners and administrators in public health to decide which diseases should be given priority, to decide which population group should be screened, and to assess how the programmes operate in practice. Although the experience of the clinician might be important, it is evident that decisions and evaluation cannot be based on selected material from selected clinics. This type of information must be replaced by data representing the normal (average) condition for all patients and the total population. The study described here has shown how far the analysis can be extended from simple medical observations based on nationwide material, using conventional statistical procedures.

The indices mentioned above, i.e. incidence, mortality, and curability, help to evaluate the significance of a disease, but further data may be necessary. The patient's need for care, quantified by the number of medical visits, the length of hospitalization and expenditure on medicine, seems to be the most necessary although they are difficult to obtain. In this context the following warning is relevant: the amount of data which can be produced today by means of electronic data processing approaches the infinite. This tendency should be resisted—the crucial issue is not to produce data, but to produce the data on which action can be taken.

REFERENCES

Horwitz, O. (1972) Epidemiology of tuberculosis in Greenland. *Acta Societatis Medicorum Scandinavica,* Supplement *6,* 233
Horwitz, O. (1973) Disease, cure and death: epidemiological and clinical parameters for chronic diseases illustrated by a model—tuberculosis. *American Journal of Epidemiology, 97,* 148
Styblo, K., Meijer, J. & Sutherland, I. (1969) The transmission of tubercle bacilli. *Bulletin of the International Union against Tuberculosis, 42,* 5

SUGGESTED TEXTS FOR BACKGROUND READING

Horwitz, O. (1969) Public health aspects of relapsing tuberculosis. *American Review of Respiratory Disease, 99,* 183
Horwitz, O. (1971) Tuberculosis risk and marital status. *American Review of Respiratory Disease, 104,* 22
Horwitz, O. (1973) Long-range evaluation of a mass screening program. *American Journal of Epidemiology, 100,* 20
Horwitz, O. & Darrow, M. (1976) Principles and effects of mass screening: Danish experience in tuberculosis screening. *Public Health Reports (USA), 91,* 146
Horwitz, O. & Magnus, K. (1974) Epidemiologic evaluations of chemoprophylaxis against tuberculosis. Twelve years follow-up of a community-wide controlled trial with special reference to the sampling method. *American Journal of Epidemiology, 99,* 333
Horwitz, O., Wilbek, E. & Erickson, P. A. (1969) Epidemiological basis of tuberculosis eradication. 10. Longitudinal studies on the risk of tuberculosis in the general population of a low-prevalence area. *Bulletin of the World Health Organization, 41,* 95
Horwitz, O. & Wilbek, E. (1971) Effect of tuberculosis infection on mortality risk. *American Review of Respiratory Disease, 104,* 643
Iversen, E. (1967) Epidemiological basis of tuberculosis eradication. 7. Application of life-table methods for assessing the prognosis for tuberculosis patients. *Bulletin of the World Health Organization, 36,* 733
Iversen, E. (1967) Epidemiological basis of tuberculosis eradication. 8. Some factors of significance for the prognosis for a tuberculosis patient. *Bulletin of the World Health Organization, 37,* 893
Magnus, K. (1968) *Epidemiological Studies of Bovine Tuberculosis Infection in Man.* p. 86. Oslo: Universitetsforlaget

CHAPTER 11

Registration in the Study of Human Cancer

Johannes Clemmesen

Based on the complete records of the Danish National Cancer Registry various categories of results from cancer registration are reviewed. Illustrative examples are given from research into leukaemia, bronchial carcinoma, bladder neoplasms, cancer of the testis, and cancer of the breast and cervix in women. Particular emphasis is placed on the effect of changes in nomenclature and coding methods on comparability of data from previous years which is of fundamental importance in this type of research. Among fruitful research fields there is mention of international comparison, evaluation of results from therapy or cancer detection campaigns, genetic studies, and analysis of socioeconomic variables and other epidemiological patterns such as exposure to drugs or occupational carcinogens.

INTRODUCTION

The quantitative estimate of a menace is a prerequisite for rational attempts at its elimination or prevention. This has been realized since the advent of modern medicine, but while systematic registration of contagious diseases has contributed considerably to efforts to reduce or even eliminate them, it has proved more difficult to achieve as much using corresponding data on chronic diseases, in particular malignant neoplasms.

There have been many attempts at census of cancer patients since it was first tried in London in 1728, but data suitable for research has never been produced by census, although they may have been of some use in practical medical planning. The first adequate data, however, were mortality statistics from Verona for the years 1760–1839, but critical evaluation of general statistics on cancer was not possible until the time of World War II when efficient diagnostic facilities were available for whole communities.

Even now, it is not often realized that the use of statistical data in aetiological studies of malignant neoplasms must differ from the application of incidence data to the epidemiology of contagious and various other diseases because of various fundamental characteristics of cancer, particularly the number of aetiological factors involved, their cumulative effects and the long latent periods.

Collection of accurate figures for cancer cases is favoured by the fact that cases not treated by fairly complicated methods are invariably fatal, so that registration of cases treated in hospitals, supplemented by death certification, will be practically complete. The exception to this is skin cancer, which in many cases may be cured by rather uncomplicated therapy, and perhaps without a satisfactory histological diagnosis being made.

PRINCIPLES OF CANCER REGISTRATION

The major difficulty in the estimation of cancer incidence arises because of the increase in frequency with age, so that information is required, not only about the age of patients, but also about the age structure of the population from which cases arise. It follows that a regional cancer registry should comprise all the cases arising within the region in question, including those treated elsewhere. However, if the purpose of registration is limited to the study of therapeutic results, and the follow-up of patients, this distinction is less important than if registers are being used for statistical or epidemiological research. In therapeutic registers the main difficulty is obtaining uniform staging and treatment of cases from the various clinical units involved, and this difficulty will increase with extension of the area covered.

According to the second recommendation of the Symposium in Oxford on the Geographical Pathology and Demography of Cancer (1950; 1952) and later adopted by a WHO Subcommittee on Cancer Registration in 1952 (WHO 1950; 1952; 1959) the following information is necessary:

total number of new cases in the area being studied (including deaths from cancers not previously recognized); structure of the total population, and of patients in the area, with respect to race, sex, and age; percentage of cases diagnosed in hospital; percentage of cases diagnosed by histological examination; percentage of cases verified by autopsy.

Although the last three items have not been reported in many cases they are indispensable for the evaluation of data, especially for future investigators, and in international comparison, where they are often sorely missed.

It follows from the above that nationwide registration will have the advantage over regional studies, both in terms of the area covered and the number of cases. But large national figures may present considerable difficulties in linkage and it might be difficult to avoid repeated registration of single cases in some places. The reverse danger of incomplete registration may be checked when possible, and by keeping an eye on the number of cases reported each year to see if there are large variations.

Naturally regional registers based on hospital records and death certificates were the first to be established; they were set up in Hamburg in 1927, Connecticut in 1935, and Upstate New York, excluding New York City in 1940. Nationwide registers followed in Denmark in 1942, Norway and Finland in 1952, Iceland in 1954, and Sweden in 1958 etc. Useful surveys of data from registers all over the world have been published in the three volumes of *Cancer Incidence in Five Continents* (Union Internationale contre le Cancer 1970; 1966; International Agency for Cancer Research 1976)

A NATIONWIDE REGISTRATION SYSTEM (DENMARK)

For the many years when only inefficient therapy existed, mortality data served as an adequate measure of cancer incidence and countries where medical access to valid mortality data was permitted, especially England, contributed valuable observations on occupational cancer. However, with increasing efficacy of treatment mortality rates became increasingly inadequate as a measure of morbidity, and when an analysis of mortality from cancer among Danish occupational groups tended to confirm English experience (Clemmesen 1941) it was suggested that a national programme of registration would offer appropriate conditions for epidemiological studies into causal factors of cancer, and also be of use to clinical workers.

All Danish hospitals agreed to send notifications of all cases of malignant neoplasms admitted, as well as of all autopsies performed on these patients, and those revealing previously undiagnosed cancer, to a central register run by the National Anti-Cancer League. A token fee for each notification has served as a reminder and helped avoid repetitions, thus saving considerable cost in sorting out and discarding redundant reports.

By courtesy of the National Health Service all death certificates are passed on to the registry. Since April 1976, the Ministry for Interior Affairs has been contributing substantially to the budget of the Cancer Register with a view to taking it over from the National Cancer Society in April 1983.

Since May 1942 this system has functioned satisfactorily, and from 1943 continuous and uniform reports have been published according to the principles adopted by the Oxford Symposium. Distribution by age is reported by five-year age groups for five consecutive years at a time, for all sites, specified for Capital Cities, Suburbs, Provincial Towns, and Rural Areas. Cases dying out of hospital amount to 5.5 per cent (Clemmesen 1965; 1969; 1974).

Although these publications may appear elaborate, they are necessary because they represent the first nationwide registration system which should be available for evaluation, even after the passage of several decades. This is particularly important since international comparison of cancer data has to take place on the basis of different medical systems and contemporaneity is of little help in reducing such differences. Furthermore, the nomenclature and code numbers developed by the World Health Organization (WHO) and now used by government agencies are revised every 10 years. This may endanger refined analysis of changes in rates, which in accurate statistics are often small from year to year and may take decades to show up properly. For the study of a group of diseases, which often requires decades of exposure and long latent periods, it is essential to gather incidence data over long periods of unchanged conditions; such situations will only exist in single communities.

INTERNATIONAL ACTIVITIES

At the end of World War II it was clear that if international comparison of cancer incidence was ever to be of value, registration programmes should, whenever possible, be established on similar principles, and based on identical, or at least comparable nomenclature. An international meeting in Copenhagen in September 1946 submitted, under the auspices of the British and Danish governments, a recommendation to this effect to the Interim Commission for WHO, and this has been implemented in succeeding decades.

In 1950 WHO established a subcommittee on cancer registration and the International Union against Cancer (UICC)—following the recommendation of a Council of International Organizations of Medical Sciences

(CIOMS) symposium at Oxford—organized its Committee on Geographical Pathology and Demography of Cancer. In the following years the latter held a series of international symposia which ultimately led to the founding of the International Agency for Cancer Research at Lyon (IARC). Linked with these efforts a considerable number of cancer registers have been established in all continents, and an international association between them has been organized.

EVALUATION OF THERAPY

Although it would be unwise to assume direct comparability of data from registers reporting events from very different medical systems, there is no doubt that registration programmes have facilitated planning and administration of cancer therapy and prevention throughout the world. Information about the numbers of cases occurring within a given district is useful for health service administration, not least as an indicator of the extent to which hospital services and their statistics meet the requirements of the entire community. For the care of single patients, however, hospital registers, with their more detailed personal information will be more useful. The same applies to statistics on results of treatment because in centralized registers difficulties caused by variations in therapeutic methods between hospitals and other therapeutic units will arise. The appropriate use for central registers in this respect is presentation of overall survival rates and trends over a number of a years as seen in the United States, Norway, and Denmark.

More detailed studies on results of treatment within a country, which may be useful to the general therapeutic policy, will in part have to contend with the uniformity of clinical data offered by studies in one or perhaps a few therapeutic units. A study by Lockwood and Stancke (1967) on cervical and endometrial uterine carcinomas in Denmark based the staging of cases largely on inspection of case records. Where basic information has been collected from notifications—of necessity on a gross scale such as 'isolated tumour versus metastases'—it may even be possible to observe previously unnoticed differences, for example the lack of effect of irradiation on Stage I mammary carcinoma, in women (Clemmesen 1977).

EVALUATION OF PREVENTIVE MEASURES

An evaluation of preventive measures using registries is particularly suitable for nationwide campaigns. An example is the Danish campaign, which took place from 1952 to 1954 to encourage self-examination of the breast, when survival for women under 45 years was markedly and permanently improved.

Since the efficacy of programmes for screening for the early stages of cervical uterine cancer will, to a large extent, depend on incidence in the population concerned which varies with socioeconomic status and age distribution, the planning of screening programmes may benefit from the accurate data of a cancer register, as in Denmark in the Borough of Frederiksberg in 1962 and the City of Copenhagen in 1968. It appears from the data of the Cancer Register that the steady upward trend of incidence rates from 44.0 per 100000 for 1943–1947 to 57.7 for 1963–1967 diminished to 44.5 per 100000 for 1968–1972 in these two adjoining parts of the capital conurbation. Table 1 shows the results for the national register subdivided for Greater Copenhagen (Capital) and Rural areas.

Corresponding observations have been made for other Danish counties, where reporting of pre-invasive stages of cervical carcinoma has been regularly followed by reduction in the numbers of cervical cancers (Clemmesen 1977). From the Connecticut Register in which in situ carcinomas have been reported for many years earlier than in Denmark, the number of invasive cervical carcinomas seems to have been decreasing since 1960–1964, although a high percentage of unspecified cases tend to cloud the picture.

GENETIC STUDIES

At an early stage of the Danish registration programme, the data compiled apparently could be used as a basis for genetic studies on mammary carcinoma (Jacobsen 1946) and on uterine cancers (Brøbeck 1949). The hereditary factor found for breast cancer was easier to demonstrate by comparison with general data, than with control probands, and this was also found for leukaemia in a study by Videbaek in 1958. A special study of twins, using a particular item on notification forms, showed that a large number of twin pairs are required for such studies because of early deaths among twins, and it also showed only a few concomitant cases of cancer (cf. Clemmesen 1965).

SOCIAL VARIABLES

In a welfare state figures for socioeconomic criteria may be more difficult to provide than is perhaps realized. However, when rent paid annually

Table 1. *Danish Cancer Registry. Cervical uterine carcinoma*, incidence rates per 100000 by age for Denmark's capital and rural areas 1943–1972 (Source: Cancer Incidence in Five Continents II)*

	20–24	25–29	30–34	35–39	40–44	45–49	50–54	55–59	60–64	65–69	All ages†
					Capital						
1943–47	1.9	11.5	34.9	57.3	93.1	93.8	105.0	84.6	66.7	67.5	43.1
1948–52	3.3	17.1	40.1	61.7	76.0	99.8	88.7	91.3	79.5	73.6	43.2
1953–57	2.4	22.2	47.0	84.5	99.0	95.3	102.3	88.6	91.3	74.5	48.5
1958–62	2.9	18.2	53.6	92.3	111.3	103.0	103.6	86.3	74.1	68.7	48.8
1963–67	3.0	17.0	63.2	94.7	130.9	122.0	107.9	94.9	82.6	61.8	53.9
1968–72	2.5	11.6	28.7	73.0	101.2	113.3	70.0	71.1	62.4	49.9	41.1
					Rural						
1943–47	2.1	9.2	25.2	29.7	42.3	45.3	38.1	27.8	31.6	16.6	18.8
1948–52	2.4	9.1	28.4	46.1	51.8	49.7	44.3	29.1	34.2	24.2	22.2
1953–57	1.8	16.5	27.4	51.9	47.6	49.0	47.9	45.2	36.0	29.3	24.2
1958–62	1.9	18.0	36.2	57.1	65.8	68.9	56.4	50.1	39.0	31.8	29.4
1963–67	1.3	9.2	34.9	61.2	72.9	71.1	54.0	48.9	42.9	35.4	30.0
1968–72	1.6	9.2	26.9	46.2	69.2	70.3	58.9	53.0	39.9	26.3	28.2

* Invasive carcinoma.
† Age-adjusted for European Standard Population.

Table 2. *Danish Cancer Registry 1943–1972. Malignant neoplasms in males, incidence per 100000, age-adjusted for European Standard Population (Source: Cancer Incidence in Five Continents II)*

Site	1943–47	1948–52	1953–57	1958–62	1963–67	1968–72
Mouth and pharynx	13.2	12.7	11.9	11.8	11.6	11.1
Digestive organs	136.7	127.9	118.7	118.0	115.5	115.1
Oesophagus	9.0	7.3	5.5	5.0	4.7	4.8
Stomach	61.7	55.0	48.8	42.6	35.9	30.7
Large intestine	21.5	21.7	20.8	23.3	25.1	26.7
Rectum	30.2	28.2	25.5	27.1	25.8	25.6
Liver and biliary passages	6.0	5.9	5.7	5.9	7.3	7.7
Pancreas	5.4	6.3	8.9	10.3	12.0	14.8
Respiratory tract	22.1	30.6	39.5	52.8	66.6	81.8
Lung	15.7	23.6	31.4	44.2	56.8	70.1
Breast	0.6	0.6	0.6	0.5	0.7	0.6
Male genitals	23.6	29.2	35.4	39.4	44.0	45.7
Prostate	18.2	23.7	29.5	32.6	36.4	37.2
Testis	3.4	3.7	4.2	5.0	5.4	6.4
Urinary tract	14.7	18.6	23.9	27.8	35.5	43.0
Kidney	5.8	6.5	7.4	8.6	10.6	12.5
Bladder	8.7	11.9	16.2	18.7	24.1	29.7
Skin	26.6	32.8	34.3	35.3	41.5	43.8
Brain and CNS	6.9	7.2	8.1	9.7	9.3	10.2
Other and unspecified	11.0	10.8	8.7	8.8	8.6	7.3
Haemopoietic system	13.3	15.2	19.6	23.1	24.7	25.3

Table 3. *Danish Cancer Registry 1943–1972. Malignant neoplasms in females. Incidence per 100000, age-adjusted for European Standard Population.* (*Source: Cancer Incidence in Five Continents, II*)

Site	1943–47	1948–52	1953–57	1958–62	1963–67	1968–72
Mouth and pharynx	4.4	4.2	3.8	4.6	4.0	3.8
Digestive organs	107.2	96.0	92.4	89.1	85.8	84.2
Oesophagus	4.3	2.9	2.7	2.2	2.3	2.2
Stomach	45.7	37.1	32.4	26.4	20.4	16.8
Large intestine	22.2	22.4	22.8	25.8	26.6	27.7
Rectum	18.4	17.3	16.4	16.6	16.4	15.8
Liver and biliary passages	9.1	7.6	8.6	7.6	8.0	8.0
Pancreas	4.3	5.2	5.9	7.1	8.2	9.6
Respiratory tract	7.1	7.7	9.3	10.0	13.0	17.6
Lung	3.9	5.1	6.1	7.4	10.3	14.3
Breast	59.4	61.2	61.4	63.6	68.9	74.7
Female genitals	63.9	68.3	75.3	79.6	82.6	77.7
Uterine cervix	31.0	33.0	35.7	39.0	39.7	34.3
Uterine corpus	11.1	13.3	14.5	15.5	16.4	16.8
Ovary	13.7	15.4	17.5	18.1	20.3	21.1
Urinary tract	8.0	8.9	10.8	12.6	14.3	16.7
Kidney	4.3	4.8	5.4	6.4	7.3	8.1
Bladder	3.4	3.8	5.2	5.8	6.5	8.0
Skin	18.1	21.3	22.8	23.3	29.7	31.0
Brain and CNS	6.4	6.2	7.0	8.5	8.6	8.7
Other and unspecified	16.8	15.0	12.6	11.6	10.7	8.8
Haemopoietic system	9.5	11.0	12.9	14.7	15.7	16.4

was used as a socioeconomic indicator, it was found that the social grading, which was unfavourable to the poor, found for uterine cancer mortality in England also applied to the incidence of cervical carcinoma in Copenhagen. A study by Røjel (1953) showed furthermore, that co-existence of cervical uterine cancer with syphilis was probably caused by exposure of the same people to the risk factors created by promiscuity rather than there being a causal relationship between them.

A similar social grading for lung cancer among males was disclosed in the same socioeconomic study. This was later confirmed elsewhere, and led to acceptance of the theory of an external cause which resulted in more direct epidemiological studies. In this context, it should be remembered that demonstration of a socioeconomic grading at a particular time and place will only be valid for that time and place. The factors leading to exposure of the less well-off to risk factors for disease may in future extend to other socioeconomic groups, so that continuous registration is necessary.

UNCOMMON TUMOUR TYPES

Cancer registration may serve a useful purpose in compilation of cases of uncommon neoplasms. An outstanding example is the Cancer Registry of Kampala, Uganda, where Davies et al (1964) provided the basis of Burkitt's studies into multicentric tumours of the jaw. In the reassessment of methods of diagnosis and treatment of rarer tumours such as penile carcinoma or male breast cancer registration has been useful, and a recent study by Lindahl (1975; 1976) has reviewed 1661 cases of thyroid carcinoma. However, it has only occasionally been possible to provide nationwide data with homogenous histological evaluation as performed by Jensen (1963) on 383 malignant extra and intraocular tumours registered from 1943 to 1952.

EPIDEMIOLOGICAL PATTERNS

While most of the subjects, mentioned so far, can be studied in a hospital-based or regional register, more specific epidemiological studies will probably require accurate information on the size and age distribution of the general population-at-risk: for such studies nationwide registers have an advantage. On the other hand, it appears that the optimal size of these registers should not exceed the population size that can be checked from individual sources of information. Large numbers are often only substitutes for more accurate collection of smaller numbers, which would allow detailed analysis and better linkage with less effort: also, the larger the register the greater the risk that its personnel may use statistical information without proper regard for epidemiological principles and as a result draw inappropriate conclusions.

Neoplasms which are increasing in frequency are often chosen as the subject of epidemiological studies using cancer registers. In such studies it may be possible to identify a suspect factor which has increased in intensity with increasing frequency of the neoplasm: the ultimate possibility is of course, removal of the factor following conclusive proof of its causative nature.

In the case of neoplasms whose frequency is relatively constant, it is assumed that most of the population will be exposed to the responsible causative factors, so that proof of their action will be difficult. The only common neoplasm observed to be decreasing in incidence without an obvious explanation is gastric carcinoma. For Denmark, the decrease is largely because of diagnostic improvement which has reduced the overestimations made previously (Clemmesen 1977); however it is difficult to exclude some real decrease in incidence, as reported in the US and Japan.

BREAST CANCER

From the crude age distribution of cases of mammary carcinoma collected in Jacobsen's genetic study (1946) irregularity in cases occurring around the menopausal age has been found. Incidence data confirmed this finding, which was ascribed to hormonal influence. Furthermore, it was found that while mammary carcinoma is more frequent among women who have never married, married women have a slightly higher incidence rate in the pre-menopausal age groups. This tendency is not statistically significant, but it has been found in Amsterdam, Australia, New York City, England, Denmark and South Wales. With this difference between pre- and post-menopausal rates the irregularity of the age distribution curve around menopause is easier to understand.

It has long been observed that childbirth, at least up to the age of 30, has a preventive effect on breast cancer, hence it is natural that data such as from Connecticut and Denmark will show a slightly increasing incidence when the number of births are decreasing. With the less favourable prognosis for breast cancer patients aged over 55 it is not surprising that in regions with an increase in average age it will be more difficult to improve survival rates.

LEUKAEMIA

Since the time of Ellermann and Bang (1908) the epidemiology of leukaemia has been thought to involve the possible transfer of a causative agent, particularly of a viral nature, and in the case of cattle, leukaemia registration has provided strong evidence that this is so (Bendixen 1973). When it was suggested that nuclear explosions might cause the increase in leukaemia rates seen in various countries, using registers it was possible to demonstrate that the increase was restricted to age groups over 60 years, and might be explained by improved care for the elderly, including better diagnosis. This situation, as well as demonstration of the 'juvenile peak' in the age distribution curves for men in Scotland, Canada, Australia and Denmark, was first found in mortality data, and later confirmed in registration material.

BRONCHIAL CARCINOMA

Between 1912 and World War II the question of whether an increase in mortality reported for lung cancer in many countries was real, or perhaps

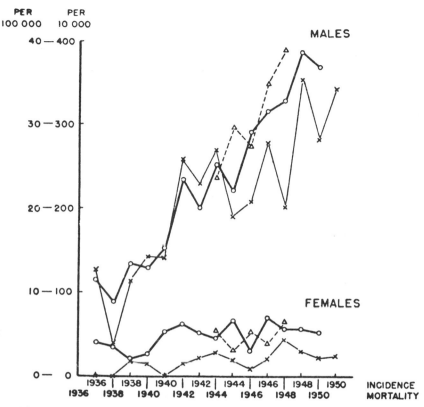

Figure 1. Incidence and mortality of lung cancer, Copenhagen 1936–1950 (Source: Clemmesen, Nielsen & Jensen 1953)

O——O   Mortality per 100000
×——×   Incidence per 10000 aged over 45 years, Central Tuberculosis Station
△- - - -△ Incidence per 100000, Cancer Registry

only a result of improvements in diagnostic techniques, was often discussed. A comparison of mortality rates in Copenhagen with incidence rates from the Cancer Registry and incidence among persons radiographically screened for tuberculosis provided according to Cornfield et al (1959), 'the greatest measure of control on the diagnostic improvement factor'. . . and thus 'evidence that the reported increase in Danish incidence is not due to diagnostic changes' (Figure 1).

Morbidity at that time came so close to mortality that by using mortality data it was demonstrated how the increase in lung cancer followed birth group cohorts, and it was also possible to predict future rates. Likewise, it was shown that this pattern was unlikely to be produced by the effect of an overall factor like air pollution affecting all age groups simultaneously. Finally, demonstration of a correlation between national cigarette consumption per male aged over 15 years, and lung cancer mortality 20 years later could only be based on mortality data, although the postulated duration of the induction period was estimated from registers. However it is doubtful that these findings would have been accepted, had they not been backed up by experience from registers for the relatively short period covered at that time.

However the use of registration data alone made it possible to perform a corresponding series of studies on tumours of the urinary bladder.

BLADDER NEOPLASMS

In 1956 it became evident from registration data that bladder tumours in Denmark were on the increase, following the same pattern of birth groups and of distribution in towns and rural areas, as did bronchial carcinoma. As it was thought that most bladder tumours, whether considered to be malignant or not at the time of first histology, were probably caused by the same agents and would all turn out to be malignant, they were all included in the study data. An interview study of all malignant cases reported in a certain period compared patients with controls matched for sex, age, place of residence and occupation. Results showed an association with smoking, although not as close as reported for bronchial carcinoma, and this was supported by a comparison with figures extracted from general data on smoking habits (Lockwood 1961).

Prospective studies on tobacco smoking effects, carried out in the US at the same time confirm this association, but in England, more attention has been directed at occupational hazards, although some association with smoking has been reported.

More recently it has been possible, by means of particularly accurate data for Copenhagen, to show that the true age distribution curves for bladder tumours and for bronchial carcinoma are identical, although bladder tumours tend to occur 10 years later in life than lung cancer. Since the two neoplasms are therefore comparable and partly a result of the same factors, the lung/bladder ratio for neoplasms has been studied. It appears that all observations made through the years in Denmark, Norway, and Sweden show a lung/bladder ratio of 3:1. As far as can be estimated from mortality data, the US as a whole also shows this ratio although individual states differ considerably, and agricultural states may even tend towards a reverse correlation between themselves (Clemmesen 1978). In England and Finland the ratios are much higher.

CANCER OF THE TESTIS

The increase of testis cancer was also first reported on the basis of registration data.

It is characteristic of this neoplasm that the increase with age after the 50th year is about the same in most countries, while international differences are largely seen in the point at which the peak appears in the age distribution curve between the age of 30 and 40. However, this peak is absent for men in Finland, Israel, for Chinese in Singapore, and for Negroes in the US.

Men in Denmark show the highest rates on record, with a doubling of rates in Copenhagen over twenty years (Figure 2), with lower rates in provincial towns and rural areas. So far, it has not been possible to demonstrate any causal factor, although it is known that temperature influences the activity of the testis epithelium considerably, and so a change in clothing habits with extensive use of tight underwear might be worth studying as a possible explanation.

EXPOSURE TO CHEMICAL COMPOUNDS

BARBITURATES

As it has been demonstrated experimentally that barbiturates may increase the number of liver tumours in strains of mice that develop such tumours, and because widely used insecticides with similar effects have been proposed as possible carcinogens in man, it was decided to examine the occurrence of cancer among epileptic patients who are subject to treatment with barbiturates in large doses over long periods. A total of 8078 patients admitted to the Filadelfia, a neuropsychiatric hospital in Denmark, from 1933 to 1962 were followed up in 1972 by means of population registers, death certificate registers, and the cancer register: expected numbers of cancer cases were calculated for each five-year age group and for consecutive periods of five years. A total of 3348 patients survived for more than 20 years after admission and had the same chief physician in charge of them from 1928 to 1959; therapeutic procedures were changed only after the findings of thorough testing had been published.

There was no evidence of an excess of cancer over the expected, except for cancer of the liver, and the inevitable number of brain tumours. The

PER MILLION

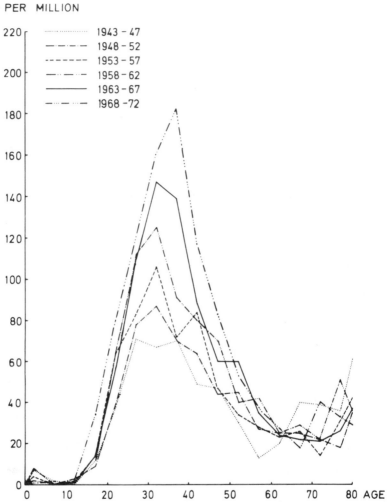

Figure 2. Cancer of the testis, Denmark 1943–1972; incidence per million men (Source: Clemmesen 1977)

liver was affected in 11 cases against an expected number of three; however, it was found that 8 of these patients had received injections of radioactive thorium dioxide (Thorotrast) in order to help diagnose brain tumours.

OCCUPATIONAL EXPOSURE

The statistical model used for the study of the possible carcinogenic effect of barbiturates is also applicable in the study of occupational exposure to compounds or procedures suspected of having carcinogenic effects.

Industrialization in Denmark took place only after World War II, and cases of occupational cancer have only rarely been reported—with the exception of some cases of cancer of the oesophagus among restaurant and hotel personnel, appearing in mortality data for 1935–1939 (Clemmesen 1941). There are two factors which tend to hamper research in this field.

First, the small numbers of people engaged in any specified occupation tend to reduce the chances of demonstrating any moderate risks, although on the other hand the regular reporting of cases to the register will favour such demonstration.

There is also the difficulty found in most countries in collecting information on people exposed to occupational risk factors several decades earlier. It is hoped that trade unions, and employers as well, may be persuaded to store records on the job assignment of individuals to allow future checks on the previous occupation of patients. Furthermore, introduction of personal identification numbers for all citizens should facilitate such checking, which has been hampered because only about 20 family names cover almost 80 per cent of the Danish people. A series of studies into cancer morbidity in various occupations is therefore under way based on comparison of the cancer register with the computerized data for all Danish employees since 1965 with a view to establishing a special pension system.

CONCLUSION

Depending on medical conditions at a local level and effectiveness of population statistics among other factors, registration of cancer cases may serve various useful purposes. Utilization of data will depend on the presence of expert knowledge on clinical medicine, pathology, and cancer research, but the ability to draw appropriate conclusions from the material will be determined by the conscientiousness of those reporting and the accuracy of numbers thus created. No international nomenclature and codes, sophisticated statistical techniques and impressive tables can cover up the shortcomings of local conditions. The value of registration of information at great cost in the form of human suffering and medical effort is beyond doubt, when undertaken with well-defined purposes, and by determined individuals. There is, however, nothing to be gained by the setting up of cancer registries for their own sake with only vague intentions in mind.

REFERENCES

Axtell, L. M., Cutler, J. & Myers, M. H. (1972) *End Results in Cancer.* Bethesda: US Public Health Service

Bendixen, H. J. (1973) Epidemiologic studies of enzootic bovine leukosis associated with the public control program in Denmark 1959–1971. Fifth Symposium on Comparative Leukemia Research, *Bibliotheca Haematologica* (Basel), *39*, 215

Brøbeck, O. (1949) *Heredity in Cancer Uteri.* A genetical and clinical study of 200 patients with cancer of the cervix uteri and 90 patients with cancer of the corpus uteri. Aarhus: Universitetsforlaget

Clemmesen, J. (1941) *Cancer and Occupation in Denmark, 1935–1939.* Copenhagen: Nordisk Forlag

Clemmesen, J. (1965) Statistical studies in the aetiology of malignant neoplasms. I, II. *Acta Pathologica et Microbiologica Scandinavica,* Supplement 174

Clemmesen, J. (1969) Statistical studies in the aetiology of malignant neoplasms. III. *Acta Pathologica et Microbiologica Scandinavica,* Supplement 209

Clemmesen, J. (1974) Statistical studies in the aetiology of malignant neoplasms. IV. *Acta Pathologica et Microbiologica Scandinavica,* Supplement 247

Clemmesen, J. (1974) On the epidemiology of leukemia. In *Advances in Acute Leukemia.* Cleton, F. J., Crowther, D. & Malpas, J. S. (eds). Amsterdam: North Holland Publishing Company

Clemmesen, J. (1977) Statistical studies in the aetiology of malignant neoplasms. V. Trends and risks in Denmark, 1943–1972. *Acta Pathologica et Microbiologica Scandinavica,* Supplement 261

Clemmesen, J. (1978) Correlation of sites. In *Symposium on the Origin of Human Cancer.* Cold Spring Harbor, 1976. (In Press)

Clemmesen, J., Nielsen, A. & Jensen, E. (1953) Mortality and incidence of cancer of the lung in Denmark and some other countries. *Acta Union Internationale contre le Cancer, 9,* 603

Cornfield, J., Haenszel, W., Hammond, E. C., Lilienfeld, A. J., Shimkin, M. B. & Wynder, E. L. (1959) Smoking and lung cancer: Recent evidence and a discussion of some questions. *Journal of National Cancer Institute, 22,* 173–203 (p. 177)

Davies, J. N. P., Elmes, S., Hutt, M. S. et al (1964) Cancer in an African community, 1897–1956. An analysis of the records of Mengo Hospital, Kampala, Uganda. I. *British Medical Journal, 1,* 259

Ellerman, V. & Bang, O. (1908) Experimentelle leukämie bei Huhnern. *Centralblatt für Bakteriologie, 46,* 595

International Agency for Research on Cancer (1976) *Cancer Incidence in Five Continents*. III. Waterhouse, J., Muir, C., Correa, P. & Powell, J. (eds). Lyon: International Agency for Research on Cancer. Scientific Publication No. 15

Jacobsen, O. (1946) *Heredity in Breast Cancer. A Genetic and Clinical Study of Two Hundred Probands*. Kobenhavn: Nyt Nordisk Forlag, Arnold Busck; London: H. K. Lewis

Jensen, O. A. (1963) Malignant melanomas of the uvea in Denmark. *Acta Ophthalmologica*, Supplement 75

Lindahl, F. (1975) Papillary thyroid carcinoma in Denmark, 1943–1963. *Cancer* (Philadelphia), *36*, 540

Lindahl, F. (1976) *Thyroid Cancer in Denmark in the Period 1943–1968*. Copenhagen: Foreningen af Danske Laegestuderendes Forlag

Lockwood, K. (1961) On the etiology of bladder tumours in Kobenhavn-Frederiksberg. *Acta Pathologica et Microbiologica Scandinavica*, Supplement 145

Lockwood, K. & Stancke, B. (1967) Survival rates for uterine cancer. *Acta Radiologica*, *6*, 1

Norway, Cancer Registry (1975) *Survival of Cancer Patients Cases Diagnosed in Norway 1953–1967*, Oslo

Røjel, J. (1953) The interrelation between uterine cancer and syphilis. Patho-demographic study. *Acta Pathologica et Microbiologica Scandinavica*, Supplement 97, 3

Symposium on Geographical Pathology and Demography of Cancer, Oxford. Preliminary Report (1950) *Journal of the National Cancer Institute*, *11*, 627. Final Report (1952) *Acta Union Internationale contre le Cancer*, *7* (special issue)

Union Internationale contre le Cancer (1966) *Cancer Incidence in Five Continents*. I. Doll, R., Payne, P. & Waterhouse, J. (eds). Heidelberg: Springer

Union Internationale contre le Cancer (1970) *Cancer Incidence in Five Continents*. II. Doll, R., Muir, C. & Waterhouse, J. (eds). Heidelberg: Springer

Videbaek, A. (1958) Familial leukemia. *Acta Pathologica et Microbiologica Scandinavica*, *44*, 372

WHO (1950) *WHO Subcommittee on Cancer Registration*. Technical Report Series Number 25, p 18. Geneva: World Health Organization

WHO (1952) *WHO Subcommittee on Cancer Registration*. Technical Report Series Number 53, p 44. Geneva: World Health Organization

WHO (1959) *WHO Subcommittee on Cancer Registration*. Technical Report Series Number 164, p 26. Geneva: World Health Organization

SUGGESTED TEXTS FOR BACKGROUND READING

Clemmesen, J. (1965) Statistical studies in the aetiology of malignant neoplasms. I & II. *Acta Pathologica et Microbiologica Scandinavica*, Supplement 174

Clemmesen, J. (1974) On the epidemiology of acute leukemia. In *Advances in Acute Leukemia*. Cleton, F. J., Crowther, D. & Malpas, J. S. (eds). Amsterdam: North Holland Publishing Company

International Agency for Research on Cancer (1976) *Cancer Incidence in Five Continents*. III. Waterhouse, J., Muir, C., Correa, P. & Powell, J. (eds). Lyon: International Agency for Research on Cancer. Scientific Publication No. 15

Union Internationale contre le Cancer (1966) *Cancer Incidence in Five Continents*. I. Doll, R., Payne, P. & Waterhouse, J. (eds). Heidelberg: Springer

Union Internationale contre le Cancer (1970) *Cancer Incidence in Five Continents*. II. Doll, R., Muir, C. & Waterhouse, J. (eds). Heidelberg: Springer

Community Registers of Myocardial Infarction as an Example of Epidemiological Register Studies

Ulrich Keil

The purpose of disease notification is to facilitate immediate action to control disease outbreaks and epidemics. Disease registration, however is also intended to provide the possibility for long-term observation and follow-up of patients. In the last decade, stimulated and organized by the World Health Organization, myocardial infarction community registers have been set up in 17 community areas in Europe, plus one in Israel and one in Australia to collect information recorded by hospitals, general practitioners and specialists working outside hospitals, as well as by pathologists and on death certificates.

The areas varied in size from 22 000 to 350 000 inhabitants in the age group 20–64 years. In 1971 all centres combined had about 13 000 suspected cases of acute myocardial infarction registered, based on a population of about 3.6 million in the age group 20–64 years.

The results to date of the WHO myocardial infarction registers have already improved our understanding of the natural history of ischaemic heart disease: they have revealed substantial differences in incidence rates in the various communities of the different countries, as well as differences in the time at which death occurs and in the ability of medical services to cope with the modern epidemic of acute myocardial infarction.

The information that about two-thirds of all deaths from myocardial infarction occur outside the hospital or are not medically attended has emphasized, more than any other finding, the paramount importance of primary prevention of ischaemic heart disease.

INTRODUCTION

In the last decade, stimulated and organized by the World Health Organization (WHO), ischaemic heart disease registers or myocardial infarction community registers have been set up in 17 areas in Europe, and one each in Israel and Australia, to collate information recorded by hospitals, general practitioners, pathologists and on death certificates.

The results obtained so far have already greatly improved our understanding of the natural history of ischaemic heart disease. The information from such register studies has shown, for example, that two-thirds of all deaths from myocardial infarction (MI) are not medically attended. This observation has perhaps contributed more than any other to medical awareness of the importance of prevention (Barker and Rose 1976).

COMMUNITY MEDICINE APPROACH TO ISCHAEMIC HEART DISEASE

Cardiovascular diseases are the leading causes of death in Europe. Ischaemic heart disease alone is responsible for about one-quarter of all deaths in males and is the single most important cause of death in people under 70 years old.

In most European countries the incidence of ischaemic heart disease seems to be increasing, particularly in males and recently also in females and the younger age groups (WHO 1973). Although developments in clinical treatment have benefited patients suffering from ischaemic heart disease this success has not been followed by any measurable reduction in reported mortality rates (with the exception of falling cardiovascular mortality rates in the US during the last few years). The study of the natural history of ischaemic heart disease outside hospital has been largely neglected. Deaths within an hour of the onset of symptoms still remain an unsolved problem for health care services and planning. Because of this the community approach to cardiovascular disease and particularly to ischaemic heart disease and stroke has been encouraged by epidemiologists and community physicians.

At the same time it was obvious that a community control programme for cardiovascular diseases could only be designed and run effectively if a comprehensive and reliable information system was established. It was agreed that epidemiological register studies provide important tools for health planning and research into the aetiological factors of the disease or disease group (WHO 1976).

Furthermore it was felt that preventive and curative programmes could be evaluated on a community basis. A community control programme of hypertension can, for example, be evaluated using a stroke register and an MI register in which the incidence rates of stroke and MI can be monitored over a long period and inferences drawn about the effectiveness of a specific intervention programme.

It should be mentioned from the start that epidemiological register studies are not passive activities, waiting for the announcement and recording of cases. On the contrary, in the WHO ischaemic heart disease and stroke registers there is an active searching for cases in a defined population. As a result register studies do not only cover institutions such as hospitals or outpatient departments but also the entire population of a defined area. The analysis of routinely collected death certificates within the register area is also part of an epidemiological register study.

PROBLEMS SOLVED BY ISCHAEMIC HEART DISEASE REGISTER STUDIES

The best answers to a number of questions asked by epidemiologists lie in register studies. Some of these questions, detailed in the WHO book on *Myocardial Infarction Community Registers* (WHO 1976) and in other sources (Epstein 1972; Pisa 1972), are mentioned here to illustrate the problems and scope of community medicine and the background to the establishment of WHO register studies.

These particular questions were:

1. What is the frequency of myocardial infarction occurring in the community and who are those at particular risk?

2. Are there any major differences in the incidence of myocardial infarction between one community and another?

3. What proportion of people suffering from ischaemic heart disease recover satisfactorily and what proportion dies?

4. When death occurs after a heart attack, where does it occur? (a) At home or in a hospital? and (b) Is there time for successful intervention by the medical services (e.g. by a physician or mobile coronary care unit)?

5. What do patients do when they experience the first symptoms of a heart attack?

6. How long do they wait before calling a doctor?

7. When medical help is sought, how long does it take the doctor to arrive and how long is it before the patient is admitted to hospital?

8. Is the acute pain of myocardial infarction the first symptom of the

disease or are there signs which precede a heart attack that might allow prediction of its development?

9. What is the influence of major coronary heart disease risk factors like smoking, hypertension and hypercholesterolaemia on the outcome of the disease?

10. Are there any environmental factors like, for example, water hardness, air pollution or certain meteorological features which may contribute to the development of myocardial infarction (Nüssel, Hehl and Scola 1975).

11. What happens to patients after leaving hospital? Do they generally return to work and do they benefit from any particular follow-up or rehabilitation programme?

12. How many of the patients suffering a heart attack had seen a physician shortly before?

13. How can those 'susceptible' in the community be detected and protected before they suffer from myocardial infarction (Epstein 1972)?

OBJECTIVES AND ADVANTAGES OF EPIDEMIOLOGICAL REGISTER STUDIES

OBJECTIVES

Eight specific objectives of epidemiological register studies can be described as follows: assessment of the incidence (attack rate) of one or more disease entities grouped by age, sex, socioeconomic status and further social, physiological and environmental variables; description of the natural history of the disease by repeated control examinations of those registered; computation of the prevalence ratio of the disease under investigation by means of the approximate formula—prevalence $\simeq$ incidence $\times$ duration of illness (in MI registration we distinguish between first, second and further attacks and between incidence and attack rates); description and evaluation of diagnostic, therapeutic and rehabilitative measures in acute and chronic phases of the disease; estimation of the medical and epidemiological significance of the disease under investigation for the population of the particular register area; analysis of the possible discrepancy between the need for medical and social care and the care actually received by the patients; evaluation of large-scale community control programmes; achieving a community diagnosis by integration of different register studies for more or less common diseases.

This last objective should be emphasized because greatest benefit will be felt from register studies of different diseases (e.g. stroke, MI and cancer) if they all take place in the same area (community) so that a total picture of the health status of a population can be evolved rather than just collecting data on different diseases for different areas of a country.

ADVANTAGES

One of the major advantages of the WHO register studies is the application of standardized data collection procedures, case definition and data recording in many communities. This provides researchers with a unique opportunity for reliable international comparison of incidence rates in different centres and also for research into the causes of these different incidence rates. By using a standardized follow-up programme the effectiveness and efficiency of different medical care systems can also be evaluated.

SELECTION OF SUITABLE COMMUNITIES

The following criteria were applied by WHO for the selection of communities for establishment of MI registers:

presence of epidemiological and cardiological skills and manpower and the necessary resources to organize a study team;

existence of a medical care system that would draw attention to people suffering heart attacks and provide full treatment facilities (WHO 1976);

cooperation of hospital doctors, and general practitioners or specialists treating patients outside hospitals;

a study population of a defined administrative area, for which accurate demographic and social data (census data) were available and which was large enough to yield at least 200 heart attacks a year (WHO 1976).

ESTABLISHING PRECISE DIAGNOSTIC CRITERIA FOR MYOCARDIAL INFARCTION

One of the most important issues of the whole MI community register programme was establishment of precise criteria for the identification of patients with myocardial infarction so that the computation of incidence rates and comparison of such rates both nationally and internationally would be meaningful. It was agreed that each centre had to adopt the defined diagnostic categories and fulfil the diagnostic criteria which were laid down in a special protocol (WHO 1970; WHO 1971a; WHO 1971b; WHO 1974).

The diagnostic categories were: definite acute myocardial infarction; possible acute myocardial infarction; non-acute myocardial infarction; and fatal cases with insufficient data. In the Heidelberg register area the last category was left out because less than 0.5 per cent of those registered were allocated to this category (Rhomberg, Mattern and Nüssel 1975). The rules for establishing these diagnostic categories can be illustrated in the form of a decision tree.

The decisions taken at each stage are logical consequences of the evidence available. Autopsy findings in fatal cases are first considered; if these are inconclusive the medical history is considered. In surviving patients however the history is considered first: following this, ECG findings are considered; in patients with some relevant medical history but without the establishment of a firm diagnosis at this stage the serum enzyme levels are examined; finally in patients with relevant history but inconclusive ECG and enzyme findings the decision is made on a basis of clinical judgment. However in such cases patients can only be placed in the category of 'possible acute myocardial infarction' and this is only possible in the absence of an alternative diagnosis (WHO 1976).

It is obvious that such a diagnostic procedure can only be a compromise but it has the advantage that subjective interpretation of data is greatly reduced. The diagnosis is therefore based on medical history, ECG findings, serum enzyme levels and autopsy results.

DATA COLLECTION, TIME OF REGISTRATION, STUDY AREAS AND PERSONS REGISTERED

By the end of 1970 17 centres in Europe, one in Israel and one in Australia were ready to participate in the ischaemic heart disease register study. These areas varied in population size from 22 000 to 350 000 in the age group 20–64 years as can be seen in Table 1. Around 1971 all centres had registered about 13 000 suspected cases of acute myocardial infarction (AMI) from a population of about 3.6 million in the age group 20–64 years.

Each area was well-defined demographically and the computation of incidence or attack rates was based on most recent census data (1965–1972). It was decided that the study should last at least one year for registration of new cases in order to obtain sufficient numbers and the follow-up period should also last for at least a year after the acute attack.

Registration began in 1971 and the outcome of each registered patient was monitored until at least the end of 1972, but in most centres registration and observation of cases went on much longer.

Table 1. *Myocardial infarction community registers (Source: WHO 1976)*

Code no	Country	Community	Population (20–64 years)
01	Sweden	Gothenburg	274 830
02	Czechoslovakia	Prague 4	119 960
03	Romania	Bucharest 4	191 760
04	Hungary	Budapest	312 810
06	Ireland	Dublin City (south of canal)	67 620
07	Federal Republic of Germany	Heidelberg	181 920
08	Finland	Helsinki	332 120
09	United Kingdom	Tower Hamlets, London	93 320
10	Netherlands	Nijmegen	132 510
11	Finland	Tampere	96 270
12	Poland	Warsaw	350 940
13	Poland	Lublin	137 900
14	Austria	Innsbruck	126 040
15	USSR	Kaunas	186 960
17	Sweden	Boden	22 380
18	Bulgaria	Sofia	274 580
30	Australia	Perth	293 860
31	Israel	Tel Aviv	121 190
50 ⎫*		Berlin,	
51 ⎬	German Democratic Republic	Pasewalk,	253 180
52 ⎭		Erfurt	
Total			3 570 150

* Combined results from Berlin (GDR), Erfurt and Pasewalk.

All male and female patients in whom there was any suspicion that AMI might have occurred, who were in the age group 20–64 years and residing in the defined registration area, were notified to the register no matter whether they were alive or dead at the time of registration. The age group 20–64 years was chosen to exclude older patients with multiple pathologies to keep the register to a manageable size and to concentrate on those who were easily accessible and still employed (however, not all centres confined their data collection to this age group) (WHO 1976).

USE OF RECORD FORMS FOR DATA COLLECTION

The duration of an AMI episode was considered to be 28 days. If a repeat infarction occurred within this period it was recorded as a complication and the patient was not counted again. A recurrent attack after 28 days was, however, considered to be a new event so the patient was registered again: because it was set up as a case register the same patient could be

Table 2. *Initial information obtained on all registered patients (Source: WHO 1976)*

Demographic information	Age, sex, source of notification to register
Details of acute attack	Place, transport used
Timing of acute attack	Delay before calling doctor, before being examined, before receiving antiarrhythmic treatment, before arriving in hospital
Immediate medical history	Presence of angina, other chest pain, tiredness, breathlessness, palpitations
Past medical history	Myocardial infarction, angina, stroke, claudication, diabetes, hypertension, whether smoker or not and amount smoked
First recorded clinical details	Presence of shock, heart rate, heart rhythm, respiratory rate, blood pressure, weight and height and source of this information

entered on the register several times. The information collected could be used to describe the disease natural history for each patient.

As soon as a patient was admitted to the register the Initial Record Form was completed. Sometimes it was not practicable to fill it in immediately but it had to be completed within 28 days. Most record forms were completed at the patient's bedside but if this was not possible information was obtained from hospital case notes, general practitioner records or interviews with relatives. The following information (Initial Record Form) was obtained on all registered patients: demographic information, details of acute attack, timing of acute attack, immediate medical history, past medical history and first recorded clinical details as described in Table 2.

Twenty-eight days after the onset of the acute attack the patient was reviewed. This first review provided an opportunity to allocate the patient to a specific diagnostic category. As already mentioned the diagnostic categories were: definite AMI; possible AMI; not-acute MI; fatal cases with insufficient data.

Information obtained at the first review, the second review and the third review covered the state of the patient, rehospitalization and complications; only at the first review diagnostic criteria were recorded and diagnostic categories allocated to the patients. The information collected at the different reviews is given in more detail in Table 3.

The second review was performed in patients with a diagnosis of

Table 3. *Information obtained at reviews in 28 days, three months and one year* (*Source: WHO 1976*)

Timing	Number and date of review
State of patient	Whether alive or dead; if in hospital, degree of recovery
Rehospitalization	How frequently rehospitalized again during the year, discharge diagnoses, number of days spent in CCU[1] and ward, whether systematic rehabilitation instituted
Complications	Congestive cardiac failure, shock, thrombo-embolism, cardiac arrest, reinfarction, angina, other
Diagnostic criteria (1st review only)	History, electrocardiagram, serum enzymes, autopsy findings, alternative diagnosis made

[1] CCU = coronary care unit

possible or definite MI three months after the acute attack. A final review was done 12 months after the acute attack.

If a patient died within the first 12 months a separate Death Record Form was completed. It contained the following items: time of death, place, whether witnessed, last medical consultation, and an International Classification of Diseases (ICD) coding of the cause of death certified either from clinical findings or from autopsy. For each patient the records consisted at least of an Initial Record Form and a First Review Form and in fatal cases a Death Record Form. Patients who survived long enough had second and third reviews.

The decision tree showing the sequence of actions taken after the notification of a suspected MI case can be seen in Figure 1.

To guarantee that as many cases as possible in the study area were notified and recorded in the register the following checks were made to trace all cases and ensure that information on them was as complete as possible. These were: (a) hospital surveillance; (b) checking of death certificates; (c) contact with medical legal authorities to cover medically unattended deaths; (d) checking of social insurance records; (e) checking the records of general practitioners and specialists practising outside hospitals (Rhomberg, Mattern and Nüssel 1975; WHO 1976).

DEMOGRAPHIC FEATURES OF THE SELECTED COMMUNITIES

Before embarking on the presentation and interpretation of some of the most important results of the WHO MI registers some striking demo-

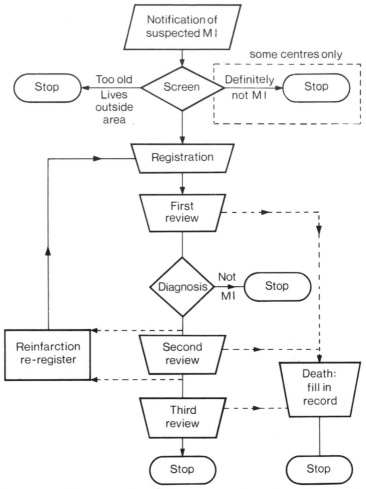

Figure 1. Decision tree showing course of action taken after receipt of notification of a suspected case of myocardial infarction (MI) (Source: WHO 1976)

graphic features of the communities in which registers were established should be mentioned.

Firstly, there is a larger proportion of younger and a smaller proportion of middle-aged people in the European population, compared with other industrialized countries like the US or Canada. Another characteristic is that the decrease in population numbers (denominator) with age does not follow the same trend in the populations of the different European communities.

There are fewer people in the age group 50–54 than in the age groups 55–59 or 60–64: the population pyramid of most European countries shows this phenomenon which is a result of the loss of soldiers and civilians during World War II and the reduction in birth rate and high infant mortality following World War I. In the Swedish, Israeli and Australian centres this phenomenon was not observed.

It is important to keep these demographic facts in mind because people who belonged to the age group 50–54 in 1971 will shift to older age groups and this is why, over the next decade, a temporary decrease in the absolute frequency of MI and other diseases of late middle age must be expected and can be explained as a cohort effect!

RESULTS FROM WHO MYOCARDIAL INFARCTION COMMUNITY REGISTERS AND THEIR SIGNIFICANCE TO COMMUNITY MEDICINE

INCIDENCE

A distinction must be made between attack rate and annual incidence rate of AMI, the latter being defined as the rate of *first* attacks occurring in a year. The incidence rate is unaffected by recurrence rate and by varying fatality from MI both of which affect the attack rate. For example, a low fatality rate and a high recurrence rate will increase the annual attack rate but have no effect on the annual incidence rate. Incidence therefore provides a more precise measure of the differing prevalence of ischaemic heart disease in different communities.

The attack rate however measures the burden of ischaemic heart disease on the medical services of the community e.g. coronary care units.

From the WHO register data there appear to be different zones of incidence rates of MI in Europe. Scandinavia and Great Britain belong to a zone with high incidence, the Netherlands, Federal Republic of Germany, Poland, Czeckoslovakia and Hungary show intermediate rates and the German Democratic Republic, USSR, Rumania, Bulgaria and Austria have low incidence rates (Table 4) (WHO 1976).

Between certain communities the differences in incidence rates are extreme. The incidence rate of MI in men living for example in Helsinki or Tampere (Finland) is about three to four times higher than that in the

Table 4. *Annual incidence rate of acute myocardial infarction (first attack) per 1000 population by age and sex* (Source: WHO 1976)*

Centre	Sex	Age group 20–39	40–44	45–49	50–54	55–59	60–64	Total† 20–64
1 Gothenburg	M	0.1	0.8	2.1	3.8	5.6	4.9	1.8
	F	0.03	0.2	0.1	0.6	1.3	1.9	0.5
2 Prague	M	0.3	1.3	2.3	5.1	6.8	7.6	2.4
	F	0.0	0.1	0.2	0.8	0.9	2.7	0.5
3 Bucharest	M	0.1	0.6	1.2	2.0	3.3	3.5	1.0
	F	0.0	0.3	0.5	0.5	0.8	1.6	0.4
4 Budapest	M	0.2	1.9	2.4	4.7	5.0	7.5	2.2
	F	0.1	0.4	0.6	1.4	1.4	3.3	0.8
6 Dublin	M	0.4	1.8	5.0	7.7	9.7	10.2	3.4
	F	0.03	0.5	1.5	1.7	2.4	3.7	1.0
7 Heidelberg	M	0.3	1.3	2.3	3.1	4.6	6.6	1.6
	F	0.0	0.1	0.2	0.3	0.5	1.8	0.3
8 Helsinki	M	0.3	2.8	5.8	9.5	12.4	14.4	3.8
	F	0.04	0.4	1.0	1.9	2.9	5.4	1.1
9 London	M	0.5	2.6	3.8	5.6	6.1	8.3	3.2
	F	0.03	0.6	0.8	0.8	2.5	3.7	1.0
10 Nijmegen	M	0.3	2.4	3.7	7.6	9.1	11.8	2.8
	F	0.1	0.5	0.3	0.9	2.0	4.4	0.7
11 Tampere	M	0.2	2.4	4.4	7.4	9.2	15.9	3.2
	F	0.0	0.0	0.7	0.7	1.9	4.3	0.7
12 Warsaw	M	0.3	1.7	2.8	4.6	5.4	7.4	2.0
	F	0.03	0.2	0.9	1.3	1.8	3.0	0.7
13 Lublin	M	0.2	1.7	2.3	4.0	4.1	6.6	1.5
	F	0.01	0.1	0.8	0.1	0.9	1.6	0.3
14 Innsbruck	M	0.2	1.5	2.2	2.1	3.6	4.4	1.3
	F	0.04	0.0	0.4	0.7	0.7	2.0	0.4
15 Kaunas	M	0.2	1.5	2.1	4.3	2.9	7.1	1.3
	F	0.0	0.2	0.3	0.6	1.0	2.1	0.3
17 Boden	M	0.2	2.6	3.3	6.8	9.3	9.3	3.5
	F	0.0	0.0	2.4	0.8	4.1	2.7	1.1
18 Sofia	M	0.2	0.7	2.2	1.4	2.7	4.6	1.0
	F	0.01	0.1	0.0	0.1	0.7	0.9	0.1
30 Perth	M	0.3	2.5	3.9	5.3	7.2	10.0	2.9
	F	0.04	0.5	0.7	1.6	2.7	3.7	0.9
31 Tel Aviv	M	0.2	1.2	3.1	3.5	3.7	7.7	1.9
	F	0.03	0.0	0.7	1.6	2.1	4.3	0.7
50 Berlin	M	0.2	0.9	1.5	1.8	3.4	4.5	1.2
	F	0.0	0.0	0.2	1.1	2.0	2.7	0.7
51 Erfurt	M	0.1	1.1	1.2	1.9	3.3	4.4	1.1
	F	0.03	0.1	0.5	0.2	0.7	0.7	0.3
52 Pasewalk	M	0.2	1.5	4.6	0.0	3.6	9.8	1.9
	F	0.0	0.0	0.0	1.1	0.7	2.5	0.5

* Including 'definite AMI', 'possible AMI' and 'insufficient data' but excluding 'AMI none'.

† This was calculated by dividing the number of cases at age 20–64 years by the population in the same age group and by applying a factor adjusting for the study period to obtain the annual rate.

centre of Bulgaria (Sofia). Such differences raise questions about the planning of adequate health services and the formulation of hypotheses about the aetiology of MI.

Without doubt, the registers have added convincing evidence that the observed differences in incidence rates of MI really exist among the different communities in Europe. In all centres combined 11 per cent of MI occurred in patients under 45 years, 28 per cent in the age group 45–54 and 61 per cent in the age group 55–64 (WHO 1976).

DELAYS IN REACHING MEDICAL CARE

Three main intervals between the onset of symptoms and the attainment of medical care were thought to be particularly important:

patient delay, that is the interval between onset of symptoms and when the medical services are informed that an event has occurred;

doctor delay, that is the interval between calling the doctor and actual examination of the patient;

delay before reaching hospital, that is the interval between onset of symptoms and medical examination in a hospital.

Figure 2 shows the median time elapsed since the onset of symptoms for the three kinds of delay in the different register areas. It is obvious from this figure that the proportion of delay for which the patient and the doctor were each responsible varies considerably; this is partly because of local conditions and the system of obtaining medical care.

In Nijmegen and Heidelberg, for example, half the patients were examined by a doctor within one hour of the onset of acute symptoms; on the other hand in Boden (Sweden) and East Berlin the median delay was over three times this figure. In at least one centre (Prague) the discovery of a long delay before hospitalization resulted in modification of the admission procedure and reorganization of the ambulance service (WHO 1976).

TIME DISTRIBUTION OF DEATHS

Delays occurring in the early stages of MI become particularly important when the pattern and timing of mortality are considered.

About 33–45 per cent of all deaths occurring in the first year took place within 30 minutes of the onset of acute symptoms. Based on the number of people with acute symptoms it is worth noting that 20 per cent of the whole group died within an hour of onset.

Figure 3 gives two sets of information; the delay before a patient called for and received help and the time distribution of deaths. The scale at

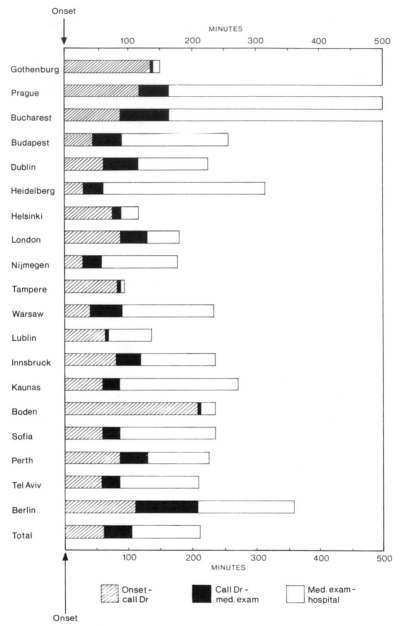

Figure 2. Median time elapsed since onset of attack, excluding cases diagnosed as 'AMI none' (Source: WHO 1976)

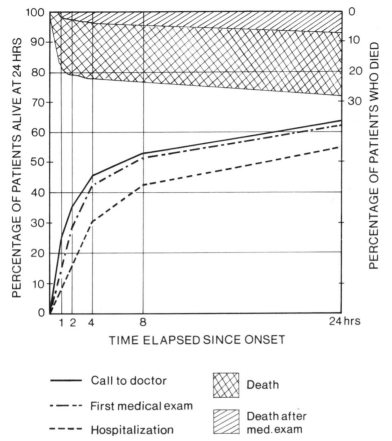

Figure 3. Relation between early mortality and delays (all centres combined) (Source: WHO 1976)

the bottom of the graph is a time scale which starts at the time of onset of symptoms and continues for the first 24 hours. The scale on the left refers to the percentage of patients alive after 24 hours who called for a doctor and received help at various times. The scale on the right of the graph starts on top and refers to the percentage of patients of the whole group, who died before and after medical examination. It can be seen from the graph that within one hour of onset of the acute attack 20 per cent of the whole group have already died; 24 hours after the acute attack about 30 per cent are dead.

The space between the rising mortality curve coming down from the top of the graph and the slowly increasing number of patients who called for medical care represents people who were still alive but had not yet called for a doctor. This space, which can be measured by a vertical line at any point in time, is heavily affected by the number of deaths which occur minutes and hours after the onset of symptoms (WHO 1976).

ONE-YEAR SURVIVAL RATES
Considering the various phases of MI it appears that the most significant phase is the immediate period following the onset of symptoms.

In the first few minutes and hours after the onset of the acute attack a large proportion of the first year's death toll of AMI takes place. After the first 30 minutes 34 per cent of all deaths have taken place and after 2½ hours half of the first year's mortality has occurred. It is impressive that the bulk of this mortality occurs before any therapeutic intervention is possible and in 58 per cent of deaths even before the patient is examined by a doctor. About 60 per cent of all deaths in MI cases happened outside hospital (WHO 1976).

From a community point of view the advances that have been (or may have been) made in hospital treatment of AMI are diminished by the fact that so many patients do not survive long enough to receive such treatment. Obviously the importance of the immediate post-attack period cannot be overestimated.

PREDICTION OF MI
For purposes of intervention it is important to know whether the onset of acute symptoms is the first symptom of ischaemic heart disease experienced. Two-thirds of males and four-fifths of females were already suffering from some form of cardiovascular disease at the time they experienced AMI. The presence of disease permits a general prediction of increased risk of MI but unfortunately it does not help predict when an acute attack will occur.

Over 50 per cent of patients who were first registered (both with and without a confirmed diagnosis of MI) experienced prodromal symptoms, mostly chest pain, in the four weeks prior to the acute attack. However in relation to prediction of MI it must be noted that these symptoms were almost as common in the group of patients who were registered but in whom the diagnosis of MI was not confirmed.

Of all patients who died of a fatal MI within 24 hours of the onset of acute symptoms 31 per cent were known to have consulted their doctor within the previous two weeks. This unfortunately indicates a poor prospect for early detection and treatment (secondary prevention) of ischaemic heart disease!

PLACE OF ONSET

The average number of MIs occurring at work was 11 per cent, with a small range in the different communities. This number also includes women (who might work at home) and men and women whose infarct occurred during the night when relatively few people are likely to be working.

When the time of onset of AMI was divided into day time and night time it could be shown that, for example, in men under 55 years about 33 per cent were at work when the infarct occurred during the day (weekends were excluded). Obviously MI does not occur at work as frequently as might be expected from the time spent by men at their place of work. An explanation is the ill health that many patients were experiencing and the warning symptoms which occur before the onset of acute symptoms keep people away from work (WHO 1976).

COMPLICATIONS OCCURRING AFTER DISCHARGE

The most common complication after discharge from the hospital is angina pectoris, which is more frequent in women than in men.

It is important that half the patients discharged experienced angina pectoris in the following few months. However, reinfarction occurred only in five per cent within the first three months and in six per cent within the first 12 months. If conditions like previous MI, hypertension, angina and diabetes were present the complication rate was increased as might be expected.

RETURN TO ACTIVE WORK

From the register data it was found that by three months about 25 per cent of those who survived the acute attack had returned to work and about half were taking part in some modified activity. After a year, however, only 40 per cent of the survivors had returned to full activity. The prospects for survivors are obviously not as good as one might expect and it appears that if a person does not return to full activity after three months his chances of doing so later are somewhat less.

As soon as this was realized active rehabilitation programmes were developed for patients after AMI. Analysis of the data related to complications after discharge and return to activity led to more intensive examination of the effects of rehabilitation and as a result programmes were modified and extended. This is only one of the many benefits expected from the MI Register Studies with their possibility of inter-country comparisons.

The results to date of the WHO MI community register studies have already increased our understanding of the natural history of ischaemic heart disease; and they have informed us of the great differences in incidence rates in the various communities, the time distribution of deaths and the ability of medical services to cope with the modern epidemic of AMI.

By the application of standardized diagnostic criteria in all centres convincing evidence has been produced that the observed differences in MI incidence rates really exist in the different communities in Europe. However, the information that about two-thirds of all deaths from MI happen outside hospital or are not medically attended has, more than any other finding, emphasized the paramount importance of primary prevention.

Without doubt the MI community registers have produced a large amount of valuable data which are still available for further careful interpretation and evaluation.

ACKNOWLEDGEMENT

The author would like to thank the Regional Office for Europe of the World Health Organization in Copenhagen for permission to reproduce tables and figures.

REFERENCES

Barker, D. J. P. & Rose, G. (1976) *Epidemiology in Medical Practice.* Edinburgh: Churchill Livingstone. pp 13–14

Epstein, F. H. (1972) Coronary heart disease epidemiology. Current aspects of research, prevention and community programs. In *Trends in Epidemiology.* Stewart, G. T. (ed). Springfield, Illinois: Charles C. Thomas. pp 168–188

Nüssel, E., Hehl, F. J. & Scola, R. (1975) Die Gesamtkonzeption der epidemiologischen Herzinfarktforschung in Heidelberg. *Medizinische Technik, 6,* 109

Pisa, Z. (1972) The WHO heart control program in Europe. In *Preventive Cardiology.* Tibblin, G., Keys, A., Werkö, L. (eds). Stockholm: Almquist & Wiksell. pp 117–123

Rhomberg, H. P., Mattern, H. J. & Nüssel, E. (1975) Das Herzinfarkt Register in Heidelberg. *Medizinische Technik, 6,* 112

WHO (1970) *Ischaemic Heart Disease Registers.* Euro 5010 (4). Copenhagen: World Health Organization Regional Office for Europe

WHO (1971a) *The Prodromal Symptoms of Myocardial Infarction and Sudden Death.* Euro 8204 (3). Copenhagen: World Health Organization Regional Office for Europe

WHO (1971b) *Ischaemic Heart Disease Registers.* Euro 8201 (5). Copenhagen: World Health Organization Regional Office for Europe

WHO (1973) *Chronic Diseases.* Public Health in Europe No. 2, pp 1–58. Copenhagen: World Health Organization Regional Office for Europe

WHO (1974) *A Simplified Registration System and Continued Surveillance of Ischaemic Heart Disease.* Euro 8201 (7). Copenhagen: World Health Organization Regional Office for Europe

WHO (1976) *Myocardial Infarction Community Registers.* Public Health in Europe No. 5, pp 1–138. Copenhagen: World Health Organization Regional Office for Europe

SUGGESTED TEXTS FOR BACKGROUND READING

Rose, G. A. & Blackburn, H. (1968) *Cardiovascular Survey Methods.* Geneva: World Health Organization

Stewart, G. T. (1972) *Trends in Epidemiology. Application to Health Services Research and Training.* Springfield, Illinois: Charles C. Thomas

WHO (1973) *Chronic Disease.* Public Health in Europe No. 2. Copenhagen: World Health Organization Regional Office for Europe

WHO (1976) *Myocardial Infarction Community Registers.* Public Health in Europe No. 5. Copenhagen: World Health Organization Regional Office for Europe

Kessler, I. I. & Levin, M. L. (1970) *The Community as an Epidemiological Laboratory.* Baltimore: Johns Hopkins University Press

Weddell, J. M. (1973) Registers and registries: a review. *International Journal of Epidemiology,* 2, 221

Conclusion to Registers

The authors of the three chapters on registers have emphasized the prerequisites of a good register—the need to have clear-cut definitions of terms, to work to well-defined objectives and to relate the findings of the register to a defined total population. The useful suggestion is made that the optimal size of the total population for any one register should be limited so that all information recorded can be collected from the primary sources of that data, for example from hospitals or local communities, rather than from regional or national compilations.

The tuberculosis register provides a useful measure of the degree of control of infection and is an invaluable tool for planning and evaluation of both prevention and treatment. Cancer registers make international comparisons possible, and enable genetic studies and studies of uncommon tumours to be carried out. In addition they enable changes in incidence of all types of cancer in different environments to be recorded. These changes may provide important clues to previously unrecognized aetiological factors. The registers also provide a framework for research into aetiology. The registers also make it possible to relate different forms of treatment to outcome from specific types of cancer on a national and international basis. There is no other way of providing all this information over successive years on an international basis. The ischaemic heart disease register has made it possible to design and run a community control programme effectively. Such a programme would have been difficult to mount without a comprehensive and reliable information system.

Registers are important tools for health planning and research into aetiological factors, and for the evaluation of intervention programmes. It is crucial to produce data on which action can be taken. The value of a register must be examined at intervals to ensure that the objectives are still relevant and are being met. If they are not, the objectives should be revised or the register closed. The critical question is: can this be done in any other way? If the answer is yes, then the register is probably a luxury.

REFERENCE

Weddell, J. M. (1973) Registers and registries: a review. *International Journal of Epidemiology*, 2, 221

SECTION 6

EXPERIMENTAL STUDIES

CHAPTER 13

Controlled Studies

Rodolfo Saracci

The randomized controlled trial is the best way to obtain an un-biased comparison of two treatment methods and over the last 30 years has been increasingly used to evaluate therapeutic and preventive treatments. Recently the method has been used in health service evaluation, e.g. for screening programmes.

Five main elements must be considered in planning a controlled study: the population; the treatments administered; the measured responses; the study design incorporating random allocation; and the statistical analysis. Three examples are described: an evaluation of a psychiatric screening procedure within general practice; an assessment of administration of high doses of ascorbic acid for prevention of 'common cold'; and a comparison of home and hospital treatment for acute myocardial infarction.

INTRODUCTION

Whatever its literal or etymological meaning over the last two decades the expression 'controlled studies' has increasingly been used to desig-nate studies in man comparing the biological, behavioural or psycho-logical responses to different and randomly allocated treatments. Here this expression is taken as equivalent to other labels like 'randomized intervention studies' and 'randomized controlled trials' (RCT) and these are the subject of this chapter; there is discussion of non-randomized intervention studies in the next chapter.

The idea that all scientific experiments involve a *comparison* between two experimental situations identical in all ways apart from the treatment under study goes back at least as far as the dawn of the modern scientific era. It became widely accepted in biology and medicine particularly through the work and the methodological writings of Claude Bernard (1813–1878), 'the founder of experimental medicine' (Singer and Under-wood 1962). The early experimental studies possessed attributes of drama and speed. Bull (1959) in a review of the historical development of clinical therapeutic trials quoted a vivid account in *The Times* of 3 June 1881 headed 'Latest Intelligence—France'. This described Pasteur's trial of a vaccine for prophylaxis of anthrax in animals in which 60 sheep were used, 25 inoculated with the vaccine and infected with anthrax, 25 infected but not inoculated, and 10 neither infected nor inoculated. Of the infected animals all those not inoculated died and all those inoculated survived. Pasteur's findings 'were immediately hailed as a triumph and applied practically'. Few trials have made such an immediate contribution or have hit the headlines in such a way. The idea that unbiased comparison can only be guaranteed by a *random allocation* of the treatments to the experimental units is much more recent and was first introduced by R. A. Fisher (1890–1962) in agricultural experimentation. The idea gained acceptance in clinical medicine and public health following pioneering work, started in England in the late thirties, by Bradford Hill (Hill 1962; Witts 1964).

The most recent development is the extension of the controlled study technique to assessment of the effectiveness and efficiency of health services at various levels of organizational complexity (Cochrane 1972). It is apparent that going from relatively simple interventions (e.g. administration of drugs) to complex ones (e.g. screening services) has two consequences: firstly, the organization of the trial becomes more difficult; and second, more complexity means less scope for generalization of study results. At one extreme it may be easy to set up a randomized trial to compare two diuretics in patients in hospital for cor pulmonale: the results can legitimately be generalized to all similar patients, without restrictions of place or time. At the other extreme it is difficult to organize a randomized trial to compare two alternative comprehensive medical care plans. In addition the results will depend on the unique features of the experimental setting, for example, attitudes of people and health personnel, local customs, explicit and implicit economic constraints, etc. They will thus have an essentially local value of a pragmatic type (i.e. as a direct input for local decision making) (Schwartz, Flamant and Lellouch 1970), with little or no opportunity to generalize to other contexts.

Such limitations should not obscure the fundamental fact that no alternative epidemiological technique (case-control or incidence studies) can guarantee that observed effects are due to treatment rather than to interfering and unrecognized factors. Therefore the practical rule for evaluating any type of treatment (e.g. a screening or diagnostic service, a drug, a rehabilitation programme) must always be: 'use a randomized controlled study'. Only if it is shown that such a study is not feasible should one resort to other methods.

BASIC PRINCIPLES

At the planning stage of a controlled study a written protocol is prepared stating in a concise yet factual way the objectives of the study and providing detailed specification of each of the following elements.

THE POPULATION TO BE STUDIED

For practical reasons controlled studies are usually carried out on selected population subgroups, for example patients in hospital or attending a given clinic, people at work in a factory or enrolled on a general practitioner list, rather than on random samples of all patients or the entire population of a city, a region, or a nation. Provided the treatments are randomly allocated this does not affect the validity of the comparisons. However generalization of the results is legitimate only for populations which are similar in all relevant variables to the one under investigation; hence the need for a careful, detailed description, with particular attention to those variables which are or may be related to the measured responses.

All variables (demographic, socioeconomic, medical) whose values are recorded for each subject in the study provide useful background information for describing the population actually investigated. In addition they can be used to subdivide the subjects into strata which may differ in their response to the treatments (see Chapter 14). Some of the variables are explicitly earmarked as criteria for admission to, or exclusion from, the study: for example in many trials age limits are introduced and subjects presenting with certain accurately defined stages of a disease only are admitted. Subjects entering the trial should be able to be assigned (randomly) to *any* of the treatments, and those for which there is a mandatory reason for a given treatment should be left out. This mechanism is essential to preserve the validity of the study, but may reduce its scope, for example when only patients at the mildest stage of a disease are admitted (Leff 1973).

THE TREATMENT

This term is used very broadly to describe any purposive intervention on the subjects in the study. It includes such activities as simply administering aspirin to discover if it is of any advantage for the secondary prevention of myocardial infarction or, with the same aim in mind, a more complex multifactorial treatment (diet and exercise plus a medication) or, at an even more sophisticated level, the administration at regular intervals of screening tests in middle-aged men to investigate whether there is any benefit in terms of mortality and morbidity. In a controlled study there are always at least two treatments to be compared. The ideal is represented by 'no-treatment', although a pure no-treatment situation may be impossible to achieve. The very fact of being given special attention and examinations as a subject in a study is likely to alter a person's responses, particularly psychological and behavioural (the so-called 'Hawthorne effect'). When dealing with pharmacological treatments one can administer to the no-treatment group a placebo, which is a preparation identical in appearance to the active medication: this allows the measurement of the net pharmacological effect of the drug over and above any effect derived from the ritual of taking medication. In many other instances, typically in life-endangering conditions (cancer, myocardial infarction), it is unethical not to give a treatment: in these cases the reference treatment is represented by that regarded as the best available. Not only the types of treatments are specified in the study protocol, but also the procedures for their administration (i.e. the 'who, when and how'). The ancillary treatments allowed, for example transfusions and general supportive therapy after surgery, are also specified in the protocol, and a record of their administration kept as part of the data obtained.

RESPONSE TO TREATMENT
This encompasses the entire spectrum of morphological and functional variables (e.g. vital status, height and weight, tumour size, blood pressure, urine density); behavioural variables (e.g. hours of sleep, consumption of medicaments); and psychological variables (e.g. score on an intelligence or personality test). Some of them, like vital status (alive or dead), are considered as hard end-points for treatment assessment while others, for example a subjective rating of wellbeing, are regarded as softer end-points. However the degree of confidence which may be given to a response is as dependent on the method of recording as on the nature of the variable. A careless assignment of causes of death may produce a less reliable indicator than a subjective scoring of wellbeing, using an appropriately designed and tested questionnaire. To improve accuracy and eliminate a potential source of bias, whenever possible, the observer recording the response should be unaware of which treatment the subject

received. This 'blind' assessment is one component in the double blind type of study, the other being the administration of treatments which appear to be identical (see Chapter 14).

DESIGN OF THE STUDY

Random allocation is the distinctive feature of a controlled study. Subjects are allocated at random to two different treatment groups; or two or more short-acting treatments are administered, in randomized order, to each subject; or units each composed of several subjects (e.g. a class, a ward) are randomized to different treatments (e.g. different vaccines). In the latter, however, if all the people in one factory or in one village are randomly allocated to one treatment and those in a second factory or village to another, comparison is restricted to only two experimental units which is not ideal. Proper random allocation as opposed to haphazard or systematic allocation, can *only* be achieved by using a well-tested randomizing instrument, like tables of random numbers. Random allocation is the only technique which guarantees that the various treatment groups will, on average, be alike for all known and, more important, for all unknown and unmeasured variables. This minimizes the chance that an observed effect is not the result of the treatment but of an interfering and unknown variable, unequally distributed between the treatment groups. Random allocation acts therefore as an insurance against the unknown.

It also guarantees that statistical confidence limits and tests of significance can be given an exact probability meaning. While random allocation is a necessary requirement for a controlled study it does not ensure that the investigation is adequate in other respects, particularly with regard to stratification (see Chapter 14).

STATISTICAL ANALYSIS

A large number of statistical techniques have been described in detail (Hill 1971; Armitage 1971; Colton 1974) for the analysis of data in a qualitative form (e.g. alive/dead), in a semi-quantitative form (score on a behavioural questionnaire) or a quantitative form (measures like weight or blood pressure). They can be applied to study designs of the 'fixed size' type, in which the responses of all subjects are analysed at the end of the study, or of the 'sequential' type, in which the response of each subject is examined as soon as it becomes available. At the planning stage the number of subjects needed for the study is calculated as a function of the size of the expected effects, the probability of detecting them and the variability of the responses. It is also wise to outline the main types of statistical analyses to be performed on the data, keeping in mind that no amount of statistical manipulation can substitute for careful data collection and record keeping (manual or computerized).

THREE EXAMPLES OF STUDY PRINCIPLES IN PRACTICE

EVALUATION OF A PSYCHIATRIC SCREENING PROCEDURE IN GENERAL PRACTICE (Johnstone and Goldberg 1976)
The aim of this controlled study was, by using questionnaires, to test the effectiveness, within a general practice setting, of a screening procedure on the course of minor emotional disorders over a twelve month follow-up period.

Study characteristics

The *population* to be investigated is represented by 1093 consecutive visits to one doctor's surgery. Patients under 15 were excluded as well as those with mental subnormality and gross psychiatric disturbances, the registered blind and the very deaf.

The *treatments* under consideration included the administration, by a receptionist, of a screening procedure (General Health Questionnaire, GHQ) intended to detect minor emotional disorders. Confirmatory diagnosis and therapeutic prescriptions (discussion therapy and psychotropic drugs if appropriate) were given by the general practitioner.

The people screened were to be contrasted with those not screened (see under study design) with respect to a number of *responses*, which included a further interview and GHQ given after twelve months, a record of the number and type of consultations during the follow-up year and a record of new overt cases of disorders occurring during the same period.

According to the *study design* all those who attended consecutively were first administered the GHQ, followed by a routine interview with the GP who did not know the results of the GHQ. At this point he could only distinguish the overtly disturbed patients (i.e. 'conspicuous psychiatric morbidity'). The results on the GHQ of those subjects with an odd entry number were then disclosed to the GP who, using this new information supplemented by a discussion with the patient, identified a group of 60 patients (group A) with latent disorders ('hidden psychiatric morbidity') to be given therapeutic treatment. The 'untreated' (i.e. not given therapy) controls were represented by the patients with an even

Table 1. *Duration of initial episode and total duration of disturbance during the survey year, for the three groups of patients: mean±S.D.*

Group	No.	Mean duration of initial episode (months)	Total duration of psychiatric disturbance in survey year (months)
A (treated)	60	2.8±3.2	4.2±3.4
B (untreated)	59	5.3±4.0	6.3±4.4
C (treated)	60	2.9±3.4	4.4±3.5
A v B		$t = 3.4$ (P <0.01)	$t = $ (P < 0.01)
C v B		$t = 5.2$ (P < 0.01)	$t = $ (P < 0.01)

entry number. They included a group of latent cases, with high scores on the GHQ, who remained undiscovered until the end of the follow-up period, when their initial GHQ results were examined (group B). Fifty-nine patients were included in this group. A second control group (group C), also to be treated, was formed by picking 60 patients at random from the conspicuous morbidity cases.

Main results

Among the controls 13 new cases of overt disturbance, most of them mild, occurred during the 12-month follow-up period, while none were reported among the screened subjects (P < 0.001, a statistically significant difference). In addition to this indication of benefit the cases detected through screening and who received treatment had a significantly shorter mean duration of the initial episode and of the total duration of psychiatric disturbance in the survey year than the untreated cases. These shorter duration disturbances were, however, very similar to those of the subjects first diagnosed (and treated) at the overt stage (Table 1). As screening presumably allows earlier detection, this may indicate a shortening of the total duration of disorders in patients identified by screening. The total amount of consultations was similar in all three groups with significantly more consultations (P < 0.01) of the psychiatric type in the two treated groups (49 per cent and 26 per cent) than in the untreated ones (11 per cent).

Comments

Among the various criteria (Wilson and Jungner 1968; Nuffield Provincial Hospitals Trust 1968) needed to evaluate a screening procedure (in fact a screening procedure plus a confirmatory diagnosis plus the appropriate treatment) two are particularly relevant to a controlled study.

The first is the rates at which, in screened and unscreened sections of the population, new cases occur during the follow-up period: these cases may be represented by new occurrences of the screened condition itself (e.g. carcinoma of the cervix) or by a related sequel which may represent an even more meaningful end-point (e.g. death from cancer of the cervix, which is the primary event to be avoided).

The second criterion needed to evaluate a screening procedure is the course of the disease in subjects diagnosed and treated at the overt stage contrasted with those discovered earlier through the screening mechanism.

With both these criteria there seems to be an indication of some benefit derived from such screening in the short term (e.g. 12 months). But the validity of this result must be judged with caution in view of the following limitations of the study. A systematic allocation procedure, based on even and odd entry numbers was used: even in otherwise good studies this method is still common; it is certainly better than a haphazard procedure, but it is not necessarily equivalent to random allocation.

Also, few details were provided on the comparability of the three groups in terms of sex, age, severity of disease, etc, and neither was there a blind assessment of the subjects' responses. Finally, and most important, the adverse effects of screening, particularly in the case of a psychiatric screening, inducement of subjects into a sick role and/or fixation and labelling in it, were not considered.

EVALUATION OF ASCORBIC ACID IN THE PREVENTION OF THE COMMON COLD (Saracci, Bardelli and Mariani, unpublished data)
The aim of this study was to assess the effectiveness of high daily doses of ascorbic acid in preventing the occurrence of the 'common cold'.

Study characteristics
The *population* to be investigated was composed of soldiers serving in a parachute regiment. A total of 446 men volunteered to participate in the trial.

The *treatments* consisted of daily self-administration of ascorbic acid, prepared in a sweet effervescent form (10 g in small sealed envelopes). Three types of formulae, identical in appearance, were prepared containing 50 mg (about the normal daily dietary intake), 1 g and 4 g of ascorbic acid. A box of envelopes sufficient for 30 days was given to each participant on entry to the trial, and again at the one month interview.

The *responses* to be measured included an interview at the end of the first and second months. The presence or absence of general symptoms (headaches, chills, 'rheumatic' pain, fever), respiratory symptoms (nasal obstruction or catarrh, cough, sore throat), intestinal symptoms (gastric pain, nausea, diarrhoea, vomiting) during the previous month were recorded. A daily note of these symptoms was also recorded on a form by the subject, and used as a check.

According to the *design* of the study the subjects were to be randomly allocated (using random numbers) to one of the three treatments. A record was kept for each subject of age, type of service, number of years in the service, smoking habits, frequency of 'common cold' in the previous year, presence of any general, respiratory or intestinal symptoms at the time of entry to the study. The study was of the double-blind type, both subject and interviewers being unaware of which of the three treatments had been allocated to each subject.

Main results

A total of 148 subjects were allocated to the 50 mg group, 149 to the 1 g group and 149 to the 4 g group. A series of tabulations, in which the distribution of the subjects by age, smoking habits, type and length of service, frequency of 'common cold' in the previous year, and presence of symptoms at the time of entry into the study, were compared in the three treatment groups: they did not show any statistically significant difference. In the two months of the study a number of subjects dropped out of the trial: these were equally distributed among the three treatment groups and the reasons for dropping out (e.g. spontaneous discontinuation, transfer to another regiment) were also evenly distributed. Table 2 further illustrates the study results. The symptoms have been grouped into four main categories and it appears that no differences can be detected between the three treatment groups at the first monthly interview. Similar results were obtained at the second monthly interview, and also when the subjects were sub-classified by age, smoking habits and other baseline characteristics.

Comments

This study suggests that daily high doses of ascorbic acid are no more effective than normal dietary intake in preventing the occurrence of 'common colds'. However the following reservations should be mentioned:

(a) there was no guarantee (apart from statements made by the subjects and a check on the boxes at the monthly interview) that the subjects had

Table 2. *Distribution of subjects by symptoms at the first monthly interview*

Percentage of subjects with:	Treatments			Total
	50 mg	1 g	4 g	
No symptoms	26.3	26.3	25.9	26.2
Simple respiratory symptoms	41.7	34.7	30.6	35.6
Respiratory symptoms plus general symptoms	19.4	17.9	25.0	20.9
Other symptoms	12.6	21.1	18.6	17.3
	100.0	100.0	100.0	100.0
	(103)	(95)	(107)	(305)

Chi-square (6 d.f.): 5.37 (0.5 < P < 0.7)

actually taken the medication, rather than thrown it away or exchanged it with colleagues;

(b) 'soft' end-points, namely interview data supplemented by records kept by the subjects were used;

(c) and the population was essentially composed of healthy, young men.

These factors might well have obscured any beneficial effect of ascorbic acid, particularly if it was small.

EVALUATION OF HOME VERSUS HOSPITAL CARE FOR MYOCARDIAL INFARCTION PATIENTS (Mather et al 1971; Mather et al 1976)
The aim of the study was to compare the effect on survival of treatment at home with treatment in a hospital coronary care unit for acute myocardial infarction patients.

Study characteristics

The *population* chosen for this investigation was that under the care of 458 general practitioners in four areas of England who agree to participate. Enrolment of patients started between October 1966 and April 1968 in the four areas. Every patient suspected to have had a myocardial infarction (MI) in the last 48 hours was admitted, but those not fulfilling the diagnostic criteria were later excluded. Diagnostic criteria for MI included:

(a) ECG changes for 'very probable' MI (WHO 1959 criteria) developing during the episode;

(b) or ECG changes of 'possible' MI associated with elevation of appropriate enzymes (lactic acid dehydrogenase and serum glutamic acid phosphatase) in the absence of obvious causes;

(c) or autopsy evidence of recent MI or coronary occlusion.

The diagnostic assessment was made at the hospital. For patients staying at home, at least three ECGs were recorded and two blood specimens taken. Women and patients over 70 were excluded from the trial. The *treatments* to be administered consisted of:

(a) home treatment, as practised under GP direction;

(b) hospital treatment in coronary care units (one in each area) for a minimum of 48 hours before transfer to an adjacent medical ward—all four units adopted uniform guidelines for treatment.

Study design

Patients who could either be allocated to home or hospital treatment, were assigned by opening a sealed envelope containing the indication for treatment (e.g. home or hospital), the contents of the envelope had been determined by a random procedure. The main *response* to be measured was survival.

Main results

A total of 1895 patients entered the trial, of whom 1294 (68 per cent) were sent to hospital electively or mandatorily and 151 (8 per cent) chose to remain at home. Thus 450 were available for the randomized groups, which included 226 allocated to home and 224 to hospital: the percentage of patients randomly allocated, varied from 21 per cent to 25 per cent in the four areas. A series of tables was constructed to check the comparability of the two randomized groups with respect to age, history of angina and/or infarction, history of hypertension and/or diabetes and interval from onset of symptoms to first receipt of medical care: no appreciable differences were found. The survival experience is shown in Figure 1 which indicates a slightly (but not significantly) better survival in the home treated group, the difference at 330 days being 6 per cent in favour of home (with 95 per cent confidence limits of 14.5 per cent in favour of home and 1.3 per cent in favour of hospital). Greater age and low initial blood pressure seem to accentuate this difference.

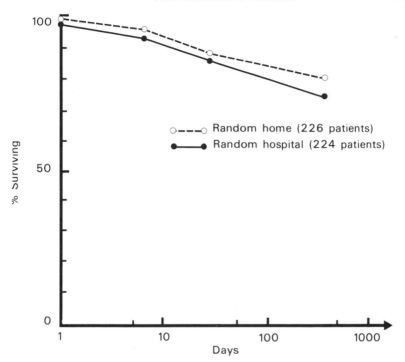

Figure 1. Survival after myocardial infarction in randomly allocated patients

Comments

This trial shows, through a valid comparison of two randomly allocated treatments, that in a purposively selected subgroup of acute MI patients (i.e. those not electively sent to hospital or kept at home) home treatment is equivalent to, or perhaps better than, treatment in a coronary care unit. For the purposes of generalization the key question is: is this conclusion applicable to all MI patients and, if not, to which set of identifiable patients does it apply? This question cannot be answered definitely on the basis of the information presented. First, the two randomized groups do not fully reflect the characteristics of all the other patients in the trial. They are broadly similar to those electively going to hospital or electively kept at home, particularly in the distribution of the intervals between onset of symptoms and first medical examination, but elective hospital subjects had a slightly higher proportion of younger patients as well as a higher proportion of patients with signs of heart failure or initial hypertension. The elective hospital group also had a higher fatality, and the elective home group a lower one, than the two randomized groups. Second, although the criteria for elective assignment to home or hospital were explicit in general terms (see above) their application was left to the judgement of the individual doctor. Different general practitioners faced with exactly the same cases would probably have made a different selection. A further point is that the opportunities for and quality of home treatment are likely to be influenced by features (economic, social and educational) of the areas where the trial was conducted.

All these factors limit the scope for generalization of the trial results. A more detailed delineation of the allocation criteria and/or a different study design (e.g. one in which subjects are *first* randomly allocated to home or hospital treatment, with some then being electively removed from the original treatment) would have helped to overcome this limitation. However, this study provides:

(a) the only sound piece of evidence available today on an important (medically and economically) issue, namely home or hospital treatment for MI;

(b) a definite criterion for decision making within the operational setting in which it was carried out. It would be useful if investigators in different locations would join in the effort to assess through controlled studies the comparative value of hospital coronary care and home care for MI.

CONCLUSIONS

It must be appreciated that not every controlled study is automatically a good one. If, for example, it is medically ill-conceived it will simply be useless, but other things being equal its 'non-controlled' counterpart would be even worse. In the near future we can welcome, as a sign of scientific maturity, the expansion of the controlled study technique in the evaluation of health services. Studies like the WHO clofibrate trial (on primary prevention of coronary disease) or the WHO multifactorial trial on hypertension control are encouraging developments in this direction within Europe. However if the results are not to remain sterile it is urgent that the meaning and special merits of controlled studies for health services evaluation and planning become appreciated not only in medical circles but particularly among health policy makers.

REFERENCES

Armitage, P. (1971) *Statistical Methods in Medical Research.* Oxford: Blackwell

Bull, J. P. (1959) The historical development of clinical therapeutic trials. *Journal of Chronic Diseases, 10,* 28

Cochrane, A. L. (1972) *Effectiveness and Efficiency.* London: Nuffield Provincial Hospitals Trust

Colton, T. (1974) *Statistics in Medicine.* Boston: Little Brown

Hill, A. B. (1962) *Statistical Methods in Clinical and Preventive Medicine.* Edinburgh: Churchill Livingstone

Hill, A. B. (1971) *Principles of Medical Statistics, 9th Ed.* London: The Lancet

Johnstone, A. & Goldberg, D. (1976) Psychiatric screening in general practice. *Lancet, 1,* 605

Leff, J. P. (1973) Influence of selection of patients on results of clinical trials. *British Medical Journal, 4,* 156

Mather, H. G., Pearson, N. G., Read, K. L. Q., Shaw, D. B., Steed, G. R., Thorne, M. G., Jones, S., Guerrier, C. J., Eraut, C. D., McHugh, P. M., Chowdhury, N. R., Jafary, M. H. & Wallace, T. J. (1971) Acute myocardial infarction: home and hospital treatment. *British Medical Journal, 3,* 334

Mather, H. G., Morgan, D. C., Pearson, N. G., Read, K. L. Q., Shaw, D. B., Steed, G. R., Thorne, M. G., Lawrence, C. J. & Riley, I. S. (1976) Myocardial infarction: a comparison between home and hospital care for patients. *British Medical Journal, 1,* 925

Nuffield Provincial Hospitals Trust (1968) *Screening in Medical Care.* London: Oxford University Press

Schwartz, D., Flamant, R. & Lellouch, J. (1970) *L'Essai Thérapeutique Chez l'Homme.* Paris: Flammarion

Singer, C. S. & Underwood, E. A. (1962) *A Short History of Medicine* (2nd Ed). Oxford: Clarendon Press

Wilson, J. M. G. & Jungner, G. (1968) *Principles and Practice of Screening for Diseases.* Geneva: World Health Organization

Witts, L. J. (1964) *Medical Surveys and Clinical Trials.* London: Oxford University Press

SUGGESTED TEXTS FOR BACKGROUND READING

Cochrane, A. L. (1972) *Effectiveness and Efficiency.* London: Nuffield Provincial Hospitals Trust

Hill, A. B. (1962) *Statistical Methods in Clinical and Preventive Medicine.* Edinburgh: Churchill Livingstone

Schwartz, D., Flamant, R. & Lellouch, J. (1970) *L'Essai Thérapeutique Chez l'Homme.* Paris: Flammarion

Witts, L. J. (1964) *Medical Surveys and Clinical Trials.* London: Oxford University Press

CHAPTER 14 ·

Experimental Studies

Jean Weddell

An attempt is made to define the essentials of an experimental study. The ethical problems that such studies may raise are discussed. Two types of experimental study are described—those employing non-randomized and randomized controls respectively —examples are given. The sampling techniques of random allocation, stratified sampling and cluster sampling are described and illustrated. This is followed by a section on study design, including cross-over trials, factorial experiments and sequential trials. The importance of proper organization of the study is stressed. The need for and problems of multicentre trials are discussed. The final section gives examples of the applications of experimental studies to problems of health care: vaccine trials, the measurement of economic as well as clinical outcome, the assessment of patient and practitioner satisfaction, an illustration of a long-term controlled trial, and community-based studies. The importance of experimental studies in attempts to improve the planning and delivery of health care is emphasized.

INTRODUCTION

The essence of an experimental study is the comparison of outcome in groups of people given treatment or care of differing types, or exposed to a factor which may play an important part in the aetiology of a condition. The groups compared in this way need to resemble each other closely, except for the treatment, care or possible aetiological factor being studied. Any difference in outcome is then likely to be due to the treatment, care or aetiological factor being compared, rather than to other variables. If those in the study are representative of the total population from which they have been drawn, the findings can be applied to that total population. If those studied are unrepresentative, the findings apply only to them and others like them.

Since the end of the nineteenth century the tempo and pattern of disease in the more developed countries has altered dramatically. This change is now taking place even more rapidly in the developing countries. Instead of being acutely ill and either making a complete recovery or dying within a few days from such conditions as typhoid or puerperal sepsis, people live for years with diseases such as chronic bronchitis or ischaemic heart disease. This change has been reflected in the type and scope of experimental studies. The early trials focused on the specific problems of, for example, drug treatment of pulmonary tuberculosis (Medical Research Council 1948). Much more common today are long-term and highly complex studies of the aetiology, treatment and care of chronic conditions.

THE ETHICS OF EXPERIMENTAL STUDIES

A case-control study of aetiological factors, such as the relationship of smoking with lung cancer, which is based on the comparison of smoking in cases of lung cancer and controls, does not as a rule pose any ethical problems. The ethical problems that have to be considered when the experimenter plays an active part, and allocates patients at random to different treatment or care groups, are more difficult to resolve. When real doubt exists as to which is the better of two or more forms of care, then a trial is needed, provided the question is of sufficient importance to merit an answer. The ethics of such a trial have then to be considered. It must be safe for any of the patients to be allocated at random to any of the types of care being studied. If a group of patients cannot safely be allocated to one of the treatments, then this is stated in the protocol and these patients are excluded from the trial.

The Declaration of Helsinki (1964) and the statement by the Medical Research Council of Great Britain (1962–1963) on responsibility in investigations on human subjects give clear recommendations for investigators carrying out medical research. The observance of these recommendations ensures that medical research is ethically sound.

The consent of each individual to be included in the trial should be obtained. The patient should understand that two or more treatments or methods of care are available, that there is insufficient evidence to decide which is the most effective, that the alternatives under test carry chances of success and failure, but that the overall advantages of one over the other are not known. The patient should understand that there is no evidence to suggest that any of the treaments under test will put him to additional hazard. In these general terms consent of the patient should be obtained: the particular details of the treatments under test need not, and in some instances should not, be discussed with the patient, as this might introduce bias in his response to treatment.

It has to be decided what investigations can ethically be carried out on all admitted to the trial; these range from routine haematological or biochemical tests to the mildly unpleasant though normally safe investigations such as intravenous pyelography, to those that carry a definite risk, such as cardiac catheterization. A second guide is whether the investigator would be prepared to allow the tests to be carried out on his nearest and dearest if he had the same condition.

There may be only one opportunity afforded to investigators to put different forms of investigation or treatment to the test. A classic example of this was the need to test the effectiveness of cervical cytology in reducing mortality from cancer of the cervix. The early findings of cytological screening for cervical cancer were accepted enthusiastically and uncritically. It seemed that at last a significant advance had been made in cancer treatment and that presymptomatic diagnosis reduced mortality. The general public and the medical profession were convinced, though without evidence, that it was unethical to deprive any woman of the opportunity of this test. Against this background it was impossible to mount a controlled trial designed to compare the outcome in the screened with the unscreened.

Black (1968) argued that the use of resources should not be controlled by pressure groups, but rather by an informed analysis of probable benefits and costs. He pointed out that preventive or therapeutic trials raise an ethical problem, in that some receive the new care or treatment, while others do not. He wrote that while it was clearly unethical, and unnecessary, to carry out a trial on a drug (or preventive measure) of proven value, it was equally unethical not to test it by the most adequate means available.

The ethical difficulties are substantial when a trial has begun and pressure is put on the investigators to end it. The objectors should appreciate that it may be due to chance, rather than anything else, that one treatment has been the most successful in the first few patients treated, and they should be told how many more patients should be admitted to the trial before a valid result is obtained. Patients may be given the same treatment in the course of normal clinical practice, but in an unplanned way in which case no useful conclusions could be drawn. Objectors must produce good reasons for ending a trial.

Ingelfinger (1975) in a discussion of the ethics of an experimental study

wrote: 'The honest physician may not make the decisions he would make
if he were acquainted with all the arguments and options. . . How much
sounder and more persuasive his advice if he has in addition an educated
understanding of the issues, if he can advise judiciously not because he
knows the truth, but because he knows the alternatives.'

TYPES OF EXPERIMENTAL STUDIES

NON-RANDOMIZED CONTROLS

The controls in this type of study are those treated in the immediate past
for the same condition by different methods. Gehan and Freireich (1974)
have argued the case for its use in controlled trials of treatment of cancer
patients. They suggested that controls might be taken from trials
previously reported in the literature or from studies carried out in the same
clinical centre or other centres doing similar work. Gehan and Freireich
cite as an example of such a trial the comparison of the treatment of
Hodgkin's disease with different combinations of chemotherapy. They
suggest that comparisons can then be made between a sequence of
studies using combinations of different drugs. This method provides valid
comparisons when the important variables such as age, disease severity
and other care given are fixed and only the treatment combinations differ
from one series to the next.

An early example of a trial using unrandomized controls was the study
by Goldberger and colleagues in 1923 of the dietary prevention of pellagra
(Goldberger 1964). In 1914 it was believed that pellagra was an infection
of some kind, and communicable from one person to another. The trial
was carried out in the southern United States, in two orphanages in
Jackson, Mississippi, and in two wards of the Georgia State Sanitorium,
in all of which pellagra was common. In the orphanages and the two wards
the diet was modified, and the allowance of fresh animal proteins
and legumes greatly increased. To test the hypothesis of infection no
restrictions were imposed on new admissions by reason of any manifes-
tation of pellagra or of history of the disease. By the end of a year none
of the 172 at the orphanages who had had pellagra had suffered a
recurrence, nor had any of the 72 in the sanitorium had a recurrence,
although 47 per cent of those in wards whose diets had not been altered
had recurrent attacks. Further evidence of the effectiveness of the new
diet in preventing pellagra was found when in one of the institutions
there was a return to the original diet when the study team left: by
9½ months, 40 per cent had developed pellagra.

Provided that adequate information has been collected about patients treated in the past to match them with those currently being treated, it is possible to use this design. This type of experiment is essentially a 'before and after' study comparing the outcome in the past with that of the present. If the present outcome is compared with that of the recent past, if both phases of the work are carried out in the same centre and only the treatment has changed, then the comparison may be useful and the results should not have been affected by changes in other variables. But there is some difficulty in distinguishing between changes in the outcome of treatment from other changes that may have taken place over time, for example, in the natural history of the disease and the type of patient studied as well as in hospital practice as a result of staff or management alterations. Provided the investigators show that no other change has taken place, the conclusions are valid. These are tough requirements and they seldom occur in practice.

RANDOMIZED CONTROLLED TRIAL

In a randomized controlled trial those studied are allocated to the control and treatment groups at random so that they have an equal chance of receiving treatment or not receiving treatment; in this way the allocation is free from bias, and the probability that the two groups are similar can be calculated. The investigator introduces defined differences into the situation by managing or treating one group in one way and the controls in another. He then compares the outcome in the groups: any differences in outcome between the groups probably result from the interventions being compared rather than from other factors, as these have been reduced to a minimum by random allocation.

The disadvantages of this method are that it is not suitable for every type of problem, but is restricted to those in which patients can be safely allocated at random to either group. This imposes experimental limitations which may mean that the study differs so much from normal clinical practice that its findings are irrelevant. Only those who can safely be given any of the methods of treatment or care being studied may be included. This may lead to the study of a few unrepresentative patients, giving findings of little general use. The design should ensure that patients excluded from the trial are a small, well-defined group, and the results which are obtained can be applied to the majority given such care. A further disadvantage may be that large numbers are needed to show a difference between two forms of treatment.

TYPES OF SAMPLING

RANDOM ALLOCATION

Random sampling ensures that every person in the total population stands an equal chance of appearing in the sample, and this is the essential item in the credentials of a sample. Random allocation to the groups means that every person has an equal chance of allocation to any of the groups. Random allocation allows the probability of any differences existing between the groups selected at random to be calculated.

Talbot (1974) discussed the strengths and weaknesses of randomization and observed that without randomization it is difficult to distinguish whether a favourable result is due to chance, a real effect of treatment or other unknown differences between treated groups. He concluded: 'Randomization reduces this to real treatment effect or chance, and permits us the luxury of an informed choice.'

As far as possible, randomization eliminates selection bias, though unrepresentative samples may happen by chance, for example, all the blondes may be allocated to the same group, an interesting quirk but probably not important to the results. On the other hand, if all of the same sex or age group end up in the same group, this may well have serious consequences.

STRATIFIED SAMPLING

It may be possible, and useful, to divide the total population being studied into well-defined groups or strata, for example by age, sex or severity of the condition. Within each stratum allocation to the study groups is made at random. Such sampling increases the precision of the experiment, and is particularly necessary when small numbers are studied.

This prognostic stratification, the subdivision of subjects into subgroups (strata) with potentially different abilities to respond to the treatments, is a particularly important requirement in the study design. It may prove essential to detect treatment effects localized to particular subcategories of subjects, identified by a combination of characteristics, such as age, past medical history, and co-existing pathological conditions (co-morbidity) (Armitage and Gehan 1974).

CLUSTER SAMPLING

The selection of groups rather than the selection of individuals may carry considerable advantages of convenience, and it may save time spent on

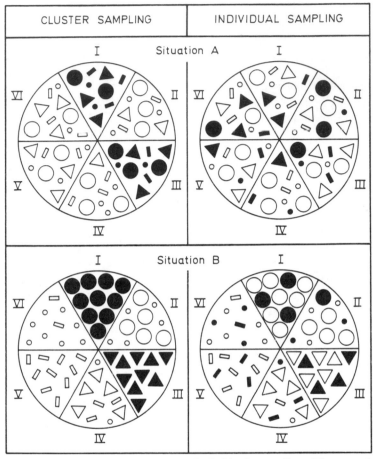

Figure 1. Cluster sampling versus individual sampling. The sampled children are indicated by heavy shading. (The different shapes—circles, triangles, and parallelograms—indicate variation in children's weight.) *Situation A*: Variance within each cluster equals variance within the total population. *Situation B*: Variance within each cluster is much smaller than variance within total population (Source: Horwitz & Magnus 1974)

field work and so reduce costs. Cluster sampling is possible when clusters are drawn at random from similar populations, and where no important differences exist between the composition of the clusters and that of the total population. The advantages and disadvantages of this technique are illustrated in Figure 1.

In situation A children of different weights are distributed equally among all six classes, so that the two clusters I and III (shaded) chosen at random are representative of the whole population, as are the individuals sampled at random from all six classes. In situation B each of the six classes contain children of the same weights, the light weights in one, the medium weights in another, and the heavy weights in another. This means that the selection of two classes or clusters at random from the six does not result in a sample representative of the whole population. In situation B there is no alternative but to draw a random sample from the total population.

STUDY DESIGN

The study design should be chosen that will provide as much information as possible, reduce bias and improve precision, minimize error and measure this error more precisely.

CROSS-OVER TRIAL

In a cross-over trial each patient is given all the treatments under trial in turn and so acts as both treated and control and each patient also acts as his own control. Comparison of the effectiveness of oral ergotamine tartrate with a placebo in the treatment of migraine provides an example of a cross-over trial (Waters 1970). Both forms of treatment were given as either green or white tablets, and all the patients in the trial received every type of tablet in turn, though in differing sequence. The colour, content or order in which the tablets were given made no difference to the outcome in terms of relief of symptoms. Such a design is essential to reduce bias where a placebo effect may be strong.

FACTORIAL EXPERIMENTS

Factorial experiments are designed to compare clinical outcome of different treatments given singly or in combination. They can be elaborated by studying outcome in patients grouped by age or severity of the disease or by some other factor. The advantages of factorial experiments are that they make it possible to study the interactions between different factors, and to measure their overall effects with greater precision.

The main disadvantage of factorial trials is the complexity of their organization and they may also be very time-consuming to carry out. Pilot studies should be done to pick out the most important factors and the range over which they should be studied. The investigators may be faced

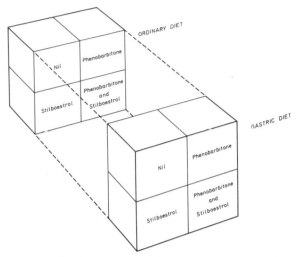

Figure 2. Trial of gastric diet, phenobarbitone and stilboestrol for treatment of duodenal ulcer (Source: Hamilton 1970)

with the choice of doing a series of simple experiments to study different aspects of a problem, or mounting a more complex factorial experiment from the start. Factorial experiments may be particularly suitable in the study of different methods of care for chronic diseases, in which the interaction of different treatments in patients of differing ages or disease severity needs to be known.

An example of a factorial experiment that made possible the comparison of eight different combinations of treatment was that carried out by Truelove (1960) (Figure 2). Stilboestrol, phenobarbitone and diet were used singly and in all combinations in the treatment of men with chronic duodenal ulcer. This use of a factorial design made it possible to test several forms of therapy simultaneously which meant greater economy of labour. Eighty patients were admitted to the trial, which lasted for five years. The trial showed that stilboestrol was beneficial in both the short and the long term.

SEQUENTIAL TRIALS
A sequential trial can be used when the investigator only needs to know which of two treatments is better and does not need to know by how much it is better. This method may allow results to be drawn from a relatively small number of patients. Pairs of patients, matched if necessary for

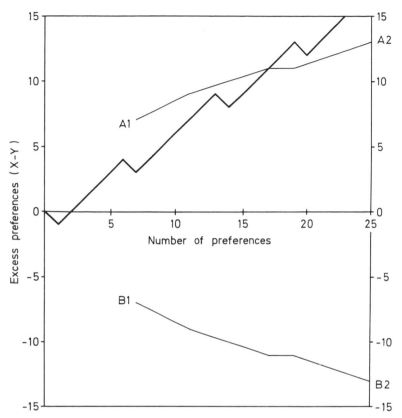

Figure 3. Sequential trial of cough suppressants (Source: Armitage 1971)

important variables, are allocated at random to two treatments A and B and the results for each pair are measured. They can show success for A, success for B, or equal success, or lack of it, for both. The results can be plotted on a diagram with two boundary lines A_1–A_2 and B_1–B_2, drawn to fit chosen values that are determined by the proportion of successes needed for A to be accepted, the proportion of successes needed for B to be accepted, and a measure of the acceptable risk of backing a loser. The lines A_1–A_2 and B_1–B_2 on Figure 3 have to be crossed before it is shown that A or B is the better of the two drugs. In this example A has been shown to be preferable to B. The technique is simple: it may save time and also reduce to a minimum the number of patients observed. The main disadvantage is that the outcome in any one patient could be compared with those who may or may not be similar. It is most valuable when used with matched pairs, but the chances of finding two similar patients to admit to a trial at the same time are small.

There are many examples of sequential trials of drugs used in the treatment of acute conditions. One quoted by Armitage (1971) (Figure 3) studied the preference of patients between an active drug X and a placebo Y as cough suppressants. Forty-five patients were studied, 17 expressed no preference, 22 preferred the active drug and six the placebo.

An example of the use of a sequential trial in surgical practice was that carried out by Vinnicombe and Shuttleworth (1966) to study the value of aminocaproic acid in the control of haemorrhage after prostatectomy. The trial extended to nine pairs of patients who had retropubic prostatectomies. Treatment was allotted randomly in each pair. In the treated group aminocaproic acid was given intravenously for 12 hours starting from the time of operation. Blood loss was estimated operatively and for five days post-operatively. The difference in blood loss was compared in the treated and controls in each pair. There was significantly more blood loss in the untreated patients—they lost nearly three times as much blood in the first 24 hours—than in those treated with aminocaproic acid.

So far, the technique of sequential analysis has not been used in trials of medical care, as distinct from cure. This is not surprising as the length of time needed before the outcome of care is known is so long that this method would rarely be applicable. In general, single- and double-blind trials, factorial experiments and sequential trials are useful only in trials of drug treatment, rather than in the wider-ranging studies of medical care.

ORGANIZATION OF THE STUDY

The problems must be clearly defined and the various solutions considered. The numbers of patients eligible for the trial must be enough to show a significant difference in outcome between the methods being compared. Clark and Downie (1966) described a quick, simple method to determine the number of patients needed in a controlled trial. It is necessary to have some idea of the degree of difference in outcome likely to result from each treatment. In practice this is not known: if it was there would be no reason to carry out the trial. But the investigators need to have some measure from past work, however approximate, of the likely success rate of each treatment. Figure 4 is a graph that can be used to determine the size of a sample that will give a 50 per cent chance of a

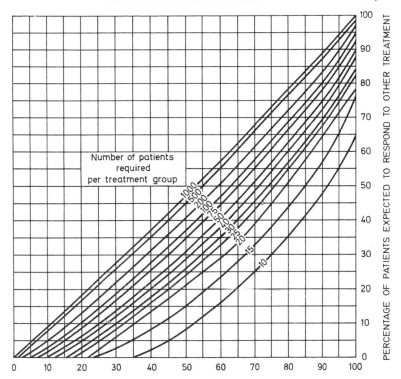

Figure 4. Number of patients required for clinical trials; 50% chance of success, 5% level of significance (Source: Clark & Downie 1966)

successful conclusion at the 5 per cent level of significance. The largest percentage expected to respond is plotted on the horizontal scale. Where considerable differences are expected, small numbers are needed. But when the differences expected are small, the numbers are much larger and the clinician has to decide how big a difference in the results of methods being compared is important or tolerable.

Peto et al (1976) in a discussion of leukaemia trials, stressed the need to compare two treatment schedules that differ substantially from each other. If a treatment improves the death rate by only 10 per cent, it is unlikely that this will be shown by a clinical trial. If the death rate is improved by 50 per cent, this is usually easy to detect, and to detect a difference of 30 per cent a multicentre trial may be needed to provide enough patients to give a result within a short enough time to be useful.

The estimated duration of the trial should be acceptable to the patients, investigators and to others who wish to apply the results. When a decision is being taken on the length of follow-up that is necessary in a clinical trial, the natural history of the condition being studied must be taken into account. For example, Shapiro, Strax and Venet (1971) have reported that the mortality from breast cancer in women 35–55 after 3½ years in women screened for the condition is significantly less than those in the control group. This result is interesting, and will become important if the same or a greater contrast is shown between the two groups at the five- and ten-year follow-ups.

The cost of carrying out a controlled trial should be compared with that of other methods, bearing in mind the present cost of caring for that group of patients, and the fact that a randomized controlled trial alone provides contemporary, comparative evidence of the merits of the methods tested in the trial.

MULTICENTRE TRIALS

Multicentre trials are particularly hazardous. The organization and long-term management of these trials is complex and if possible should be carried out by a central coordinating office. It is essential that all the centres work to common definitions, and these should be tested out in a pilot study at an early stage.

The basic treatment given to the patients must be the same in every centre, and should not change during the trial, but it may be possible to give the clinicians some freedom of choice. For example, in a study of the control of moderately raised blood pressure (Depts. of Medicine... 1973), the essential requirement was that patients in the treatment group should have their diastolic blood pressure controlled at or below 90 mm Hg, and the clinicians could use oral diuretics and hypotensive drugs singly or in combination as they wished to achieve this.

In such trials several centres have to work together, to a common protocol, for a number of years. The conditions studied, such as moderately raised blood pressure or diabetes, take some years to show measurable change in enough patients for the results to be of use. The problems raised are well illustrated by the University Group Diabetes Program (UGDP) (1970), which set out to determine whether or not the control of blood glucose levels helps to prevent or delay vascular disease in those diabetic patients not needing insulin for control. The trial was carried out in 12 centres. The patients were allocated at random to five treatment groups: placebo; a standard dose of tolbutamide (1.5 g/day); a standard dose of insulin; a variable dose of insulin; or a standard dose of phenformin (100 mg/day). After 8½ years follow-up: 'The findings of the study indicate that the combination of diet and tolbutamide therapy is no more effective than diet alone in prolonging life. Moreover, the findings suggest that tolbutamide and diet may be less effective than diet alone or diet and insulin, at least in so far as cardiovascular mortality is concerned.'

A year later the University Group published almost identical findings on phenformin (Knatterud et al 1971). The use of oral hypoglycaemic agents in general, the UGDP study in particular and the main points of the five-year controversy sparked off by its findings have been summarized by Shen and Bressler (1977). The arguments are most fierce over the selection of patients—69 patients admitted to the trial did not meet the stated UGDP criteria—and over the baseline inequalities in cardiovascular risk factors in those allocated randomly to different treatment groups. The differences in mortality rates between clinics has also been criticized, as has the use of fixed doses of tolbutamide and phenformin. Also smoking history was not included in the baseline risk factors, nor were the degree of control of hypertension or hypercholesterolaemia.

The arguments over these and other points will probably continue. Shen and Bressler wrote: 'In summary, the UGDP study has been carefully scrutinized by many, and severely criticised by some. The assessment of the validity of the study by a committee of the Biometric Society has been published (1975). The probability that oral hypoglycaemic agents cause premature deaths from cardiovascular disease remains valid and cannot be dismissed on the basis of other available evidence. The UGDP study is the most comprehensive and most adequately controlled study of oral hypoglycaemic agents published to date.'

This controversy has served one useful purpose and that is to provoke a number of people into thought about the problems raised by the UGDP study in particular and by multicentre trials in general. This is a notable advance, for such trials are expensive in terms of time, effort and resources, and are not easily repeated. Potential investigators need to be aware of the hazards.

FURTHER APPLICATIONS OF EXPERIMENTAL STUDIES TO PROBLEMS OF HEALTH CARE

VACCINE TRIALS

The Medical Research Council of Great Britain carried out a trial of the effectiveness of BCG and vole vaccine in the prevention of tuberculosis in adolescents. A total of 54 239 tuberculin negative children aged 14–15½ years were admitted to the trial between 1950 and 1952. They were allocated at random to two control groups, and to two treatment groups, one being vaccinated with BCG and the other with vole vaccine. The reduction in the incidence of tuberculosis in those given BCG was 83 per cent, and in those given vole vaccine was 87 per cent by 1960, at a mean follow-up of 8.8 years.

This trial established the effectiveness of the two vaccines in reducing the incidence of tuberculosis in adolescents, and such vaccination was then given to most schoolchildren in Great Britain until the incidence of tuberculosis fell to such a low level that the costs outweighed the benefits.

THE MEASUREMENT OF ECONOMIC AS WELL AS CLINICAL OUTCOME

Piachaud and Weddell (1972) compared not only the clinical outcome of treating varicose veins by inpatient surgery and outpatient injection–compression sclerotherapy, but also the costs of the respective treatments. There was found to be no difference in the results of treatment at three-year follow-up. Consequently, on the basis that surgical treatment is more expensive than injection–compression sclerotherapy, the authors were able to recommend the latter treatment as being more cost-effective.

A TRIAL MEASURING PATIENT AND PRACTITIONER SATISFACTION

Adler et al (1974) have extended the method of controlled comparison even further in a randomized controlled trial of early discharge for inguinal hernia and varicose veins. In addition to the clinical outcome and cost measured by Piachaud and Weddell, the satisfaction of the patient, his family, the practitioner and the district nurse were also measured. Some of the factors involved, such as length of convalescence, amount of work generated for district nurses and for general practitioners, are relatively easy to measure. The comparison of attitudes to different methods of medical care is, however, subjective and their importance is difficult to evaluate.

A LONG-TERM CONTROLLED TRIAL

D'Souza, Swan and Shannon (1976) have cast doubts on the cost-effectiveness of screening for hypertension in general practice, in a study carried out on samples from the populations of two general practices in south-east England, over a period of seven years. No significant difference in blood pressure levels was observed between the control and screened groups. Over 95 per cent of the new hypertensives discovered in the comparative screening of the control group had visited their general practitioner during the previous five years. These two findings suggest, firstly, that screening generates little effective therapeutic intervention; and, secondly, that case-finding is more cost-effective than screening.

COMMUNITY-BASED STUDIES

Elwood, Waters and Sweetnam (1971) have reported two-way community-based studies of the haematinic effect of iron added to flour used to bake bread. The first was a 'therapeutic' trial of 304 women, divided at random into two groups. The first group were supplied with ordinary bread, the second group with bread made from flour containing ferric ammonium citrate. The second study was a 'prophylactic trial', in which 450 women were divided into three groups, one receiving bread with a higher level of ferric ammonium citrate, the second an equivalent amount of iron in tablet form, and the third a placebo. The trials were designed to simulate conditions in the community as closely as possible. Neither gave conclusive evidence of benefit in terms of an effect on circulating haemoglobin level.

These studies demonstrate how experimental studies can be used in a wide variety of health care applications. The contrast between the early comparative studies of drugs or vaccines and the trials comparing different styles of medical care is sharp. The former had clear end-points which were reasonably simple to measure and few in number: the latter have multiple end-points, many based on subjective measurements which are difficult to make with precision.

CONCLUSION

Experimental studies in general and the randomized controlled clinical trial in particular, provide some, but not the only, means to test methods of care. The problems that can be studied in this way are limited. The objectives of the trial must be stated clearly, and it must be possible to put the results into practice. The main purpose is to improve the care of the community and to make best use of the resources of the health service. The findings of a study should provide the planners of health services with comparisons of different types of care so that choice of a particular method can be based on the best evidence available.

REFERENCES

Adler, M. W., Waller, J. J., Day, I., Kasap, H. S., King, C. & Thorne, S. C. (1974) A randomized controlled trial of early discharge for inguinal hernia and varicose veins. Some problems of methodology. *Medical Care*, *12*, 541

Armitage, P. (1971) *Statistical Methods in Medical Research*. Oxford: Blackwell Scientific Publications

Armitage, P. & Gehan, A. (1974) Statistical methods for the identification and use of prognostic factors. *International Journal of Cancer*, *13*, 16

Black, D. A. (1968) *The Logic of Medicine*. Edinburgh: Oliver & Boyd

Clark, C. J. & Downie, C. C. (1966) A method for the rapid determination of the number of patients to include in a controlled clinical trial. *Lancet*, *2*, 1357

Declaration of Helsinki (1964) Recommendations guiding doctors in clinical research. 18th World Medical Assembly, Helsinki

Departments of Medicine and Clinical Epidemiology and Social Medicine, St Thomas's Hospital Medical School, London and Department of Medicine, United Cardiff Hospitals, and the Medical Research Council Epidemiological Research Unit, Cardiff. (1973) Control of moderately raised blood pressure. Report of a co-operative randomized controlled trial. *British Medical Journal*, *3*, 434

D'Souza, M. F., Swan, A. V. & Shannon, D. J. (1976) A long-term controlled trial of screening for hypertension in general practice. *Lancet*, *1*, 1228

Elwood, P. C., Waters, W. E. & Sweetnam, P. (1971) The haematinic effect of iron in flour. *Clinical Science*, *40*, 31

Gehan, E. A. & Freireich, E. J. (1974) Non-randomized controls in cancer clinical trials. *New England Journal of Medicine*, *290*, 198

Goldberger, J. (1964) *Goldberger on Pellagra*. Terris, M. (ed). Baton Rouge, La: Louisiana State University Press

Hamilton, M. (1970) *Lectures on the Methodology of Clinical Research*. Edinburgh: E. & S. Livingstone

Horwitz, O. & Magnus, K. (1974) Epidemiologic evaluation of chemoprophylaxis against tuberculosis. *American Journal of Epidemiology*, *99*, 333

Ingelfinger, F. J. (1975) Ethics and high blood pressure. *New England Journal of Medicine*, *292*, 43

Knatterud, G. L., Meinert, C. L., Klimt, C. R., Osborne, R. K. & Martin, D. B. (1971) Effects of hypoglycemic agents on vascular complications in patients with adult-onset diabetes. IV. A preliminary report on phenformin results. *Journal of the American Medical Association*, *217*, 777

Medical Research Council (1948) Streptomycin treatment of pulmonary tuberculosis. *British Medical Journal*, *2*, 769

Medical Research Council (1962–63) Responsibility in investigations on human subjects. Cmnd 2382

Medical Research Council (1963) (Tuberculosis vaccines Clinical Trials Committee) BCG and vole bacillus vaccines in prevention of tuberculosis in adolescents. (Third Report). *British Medical Journal, 1*, 973

Peto, R., Pike, M. C., Armitage, P., Breslow, N. E., Cox, D. R., Howard, S. V., Mantel, N., McPherson, K., Peto, J., & Smith, P. G. (1976) Design and analysis of randomized clinical trials requiring prolonged observation of each patient. I: Introduction and design. *British Journal of Cancer, 34*, 585

Piachaud, D. & Weddell, J. M. (1972) The economics of treating varicose veins. *International Journal of Epidemiology, 1*, 287

Report of the Committee for the Assessment of Biometric Aspects of Controlled Trials of Hypoglycemic Agents. (1975) *Journal of the American Medical Association, 231*, 583

Shapiro, S., Strax, P. & Venet, L. (1971) Periodic breast cancer screening in reducing mortality from breast cancer. *Journal of the American Medical Association, 215*, 1777

Shen, S-W. & Bressler, R. (1977) Clinical pharmacology of oral antidiabetic agents (Part II). *New England Journal of Medicine, 296*, 787

Talbot, J. C. (1974) Need for randomised clinical trials (letter). *New England Journal of Medicine, 290*, 1091

Truelove, S. C. (1960) Stilboestrol, phenobarbitone and diet in chronic duodenal ulcer. *British Medical Journal, 2*, 559

University Group Diabetes Program (1970) A study of the effects of hypoglycemic agents on vascular complications in patients with adult-onset diabetes. II. Mortality results. *Diabetes, 19*, Supplement, 789

Vinnicombe, J. & Shuttleworth, K. E. D. (1966) Aminocaproic acid in the control of haemorrhage after prostatectomy. *Lancet, 1*, 230

Waters, W. E. (1970) Controlled clinical trial of ergotamine tartrate. *British Medical Journal, 2*, 325

SUGGESTED TEXTS FOR BACKGROUND READING

Cochrane, A. L. (1972) *Effectiveness and Efficiency. Random Reflections on Health Services.* The Rock Carling Fellowship 1971, Nuffield Provincial Hospitals Trust

Hill, B. A. (1977) *Principles of Medical Statistics.* (10th Ed). London: Hodder & Stoughton

Oldham, P. D. (1968) *Measurement in Medicine: The Interpretation of Numerical Data.* London: The English Universities Press (Chapter 7)

Peto, R., Pike, M. C., Armitage, P., Breslow, N. E., Cox, D. R., Howard, S. V., Mantel, N., McPherson, K., Peto, J. & Smith, P. G. (1976 & 1977) Design and analysis of randomized clinical trials requiring prolonged observation of each patient. I: Introduction and design. *British Journal of Cancer, 34*, 585. II: Analysis and examples. *British Journal of Cancer, 35*, 1

SECTION 7

CAUSATION AND CONTROL
OF DISEASE

CHAPTER 15

Causation and Control with Special Reference to Rubella

Michel F. Lechat

Rubella is taken as an example of the use of epidemiological techniques in identification of causative factors of a disease. Both case-control and longitudinal studies have been used to establish the relationship between rubella during pregnancy and congenital malformations in the fetus. The epidemiological approach starting with retrospective assessment of associations between factors followed by more experimental prospective studies to measure risks is described. The application of these results to control of rubella is emphasized particularly in relation to identification of high risk groups, i.e. primary prevention by vaccination.

INTRODUCTION

In Australia in 1939–1940 a large number of cases of rubella were recorded; before that no epidemic had been noted for 17 years (Ingalls et al 1960) but in this case a large proportion of the population was affected, especially the younger age groups. In 1941, Gregg noticed the unusually high number of congenital cataracts among infants in Sydney. When the mothers of 78 newborn children with cataract were questioned about their history, 87 per cent (68) remembered having had rubella during pregnancy, most of them during the first few months. Forty-four of these children also had malformations of the heart (Gregg 1941).

These early observations by Gregg suggested that there might be an aetiological relationship between rubella during pregnancy and congenital defects in the newborn. Such an observation is the initial stage in any epidemiological approach, i.e. when the intuitive recognition of a situation which appears to differ from the norm enables formulation of a plausible hypothesis. However, it does not provide grounds for positively stating that this relationship exists without a comparable study among mothers of normal children; for it is possible that the incidence of rubella during the epidemic of 1939–1940 was 87 per cent among *all* women of child-bearing age.

In order to confirm this hypothesis the frequency of rubella among mothers of children with cataract must be compared with that in mothers of normal children. These normal children, designated the controls, must be similar to the malformed children in respect of every factor suspected of giving rise to congenital anomalies, apart from the factor under study.

By means of such studies it is possible to confirm the existence of an association between the disease in the mother and malformations in the child. However these studies do not permit quantitative estimation of the risk of fetus malformation from rubella infection in the pregnant mother. What proportion of children born to mothers infected with rubella during pregnancy are malformed? In other words: what is the risk of malformation, what are the chances of escaping it, and does the risk differ according to the month of pregnancy in which infection occurs?

LONGITUDINAL STUDIES: MEASUREMENT OF RISK

To measure the risk is to answer the question: what is the chance that a person exposed to the incriminated factor (in this case rubella during pregnancy) will be affected by the phenomenon studied (in this case the birth of a defective child)?

Only by means of longitudinal studies is it possible to calculate the risk by observing the proportion of cases in a given population exposed to the factor and by comparing this proportion with that found in a population which is similar in all respects but has not been exposed to that factor. One may then predict the risk of catching the disease according to the severity of the factor, the length of exposure time or various other conditions. According to the risks which characterize them, more or less vulnerable populations may be distinguished; and one may also compare the cost of prevention or treatment with the cost incurred as a result of the disease.

A study of this kind was carried out in Sweden in 1951 on all women who had given birth in maternity hospitals after a rubella epidemic in the country (Lundström 1952). All mothers attending maternity welfare and child health clinics throughout the country were questioned about any past history of rubella during the last pregnancy. The mothers who gave positive replies were then, and only then, questioned about the birth of a malformed child. The frequencies noted were then compared with the prevalence of defective births among a sample of mothers who had not had rubella during pregnancy; this sample consisted of women with confinement registration numbers preceding those of the mothers who had had rubella. In 80 per cent of cases the diagnosis was made retrospectively by questioning the mothers. In 609 children born to mothers who had contracted rubella during the first four months of pregnancy the risk of perinatal death (stillbirth and neonatal death), prematurity and congenital malformations (including a series of neonatal disorders for which a relationship with rubella has not been established) amounted to 17 per cent in contrast to 6 per cent in the controls whose mothers had not had rubella. On the other hand, the children of mothers who contracted rubella after the fifth month of pregnancy showed no significant differences when compared with the controls.

The difference between the frequencies observed in individuals subjected to the incriminated factor and in those who are not is a measure of the relative risk. The relative risk of perinatal death, prematurity and malformations in the children of mothers who had rubella during the first four months of pregnancy was 0.11 (i.e. 0.17–0.06) in Lundström's study. This type of study is called longitudinal because the factor whose aetiological role is suspected, in this case rubella in pregnant women, is identified first: the term 'prospective studies' is also used. Theoretically, the ideal conditions for analysis would require observation of two groups of women from the time of conception—one group consisting of women infected by rubella during pregnancy and another group of women not infected by rubella; one would thus approach experimental conditions. However such observations would not be possible. One can appreciate that ethical problems may arise in prospective studies even in less extreme situations.

A POSTERIORI LONGITUDINAL STUDIES

The epidemiologist therefore endeavours to make the best use of the experiments conducted independently of himself, i.e. in nature. For example, a rubella epidemic affecting only some of the pregnant, susceptible women.

Thus Lundström's study (1952) reported above, although longitudinal, was also a posteriori: it was after childbirth that the recently confined women were questioned about rubella during their pregnancy, initially without consideration of the presence or absence of anomalies in children born to these women. They were then classified according to whether they had had rubella or not; only subsequently was the condition of the children noted.

Studies of this type could be called 'a posteriori longitudinal': it is important not to refer to them, as so often happens, as retrospective studies since this term should be reserved for case-control studies. What characterizes the longitudinal study, be it conducted prospectively in the manner of an experimental study where this is feasible and ethically justified, or done a posteriori with documents, is that the sampling unit is constituted by the incriminated factor. In other words (Bradford Hill et al 1958) the disease must first be observed and diagnosed in women, and only subsequently should the condition of the children be noted.

If a sample is too small for statistical analysis, the data of several studies can be combined, provided they have been collected in a similar way. Warkany and Kalter (1961) combined the results of 15 studies carried out between 1946 and 1961, which included a total of 421 children born alive to women who had contracted rubella during the first 12 weeks of pregnancy: they calculated a frequency of 16.9 per cent risk of anomalies. Often it is difficult to compare the mean rates calculated in this way with those observed in controls, since the latter may differ considerably from one study to another.

In longitudinal studies carried out on an a posteriori basis a number of precautions must be taken: if the researcher sends a questionnaire to a large number of women concerning history of rubella during pregnancy and mentions that he is looking for a link with congenital anomalies, it is likely that women who gave birth to an abnormal child and had had rubella will reply more readily than the others. Hence a considerable overestimate of the risk (Wesselhoeft 1949) may be obtained. Thus, the first a posteriori studies carried out on rubella provided overestimated figures of up to 90 per cent for the risk of congenital anomalies (Warkany and Kalter 1961).

To this must be added the well-known existence of distortion in retrospective studies (case-control and a posteriori longitudinal) based on questioning. Remembrance of the incriminated factor is often related to the presence of the disorder: in this case, mothers of malformed children will tend to remember having had rubella during pregnancy more readily than mothers of normal children for whom a transitory illness that happened several months or years before is forgotten.

MEASUREMENT OF THE RISK ACCORDING TO THE STAGE OF PREGNANCY

Longitudinal studies can achieve more than a mere gauging of the risk according to the presence or absence of an aetiological factor. They also

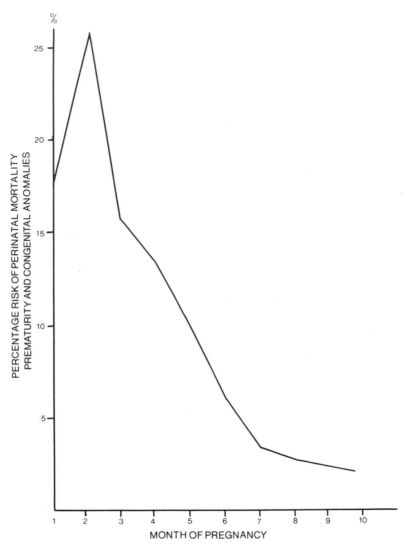

Figure 1. Risk of perinatal mortality, prematurity and congenital anomalies in 1067 children whose mothers suffered from rubella during pregnancy (Source: Lundström 1952)

Table 1. *Prevalence of major congenital anomalies at birth in children whose mothers had had rubella at different times during pregnancy* (*Source: Bradford Hill et al 1958*)

Weeks of pregnancy when rubella first contracted	Number of cases	Children with major anomalies	
		Number	%
1–4	12	6	50
5–8	20	5	25
9–12	18	3	17
13–16	18	2	11
17–24	17	1	6
25+	19	0	0

serve to measure the risk according to the severity of the factor, its time of application or perhaps other characteristics. In the study on the Swedish mothers (Lundström 1952), the risk of perinatal mortality, premature birth and congenital anomalies was greatest in children born to mothers who had had rubella in the *second* month of pregnancy (Figure 1).

Combining several studies carried out on an a posteriori basis but which satisfy the strict conditions of the longitudinal study, Bradford Hill et al (1958) calculated the prevalence of major congenital anomalies according to the stage of pregnancy when rubella was contracted (Table 1).

CHOICE OF DENOMINATOR

When observing malformations at birth the prevalence of malformations in full-term newborn babies is noted and not the incidence of malformations in fetuses exposed to rubella in utero. It is possible that rubella infection in fetuses also causes greater risk of abortion. If so, the risk of anomalies will be much higher than that found among the newborn. At the extreme end of the scale—and it is thought that this happens with certain teratogenic factors in the environment—the rate of abortion could become so high that in fact prevalence of anomalies at birth could reach zero, hence such factors would appear to be protecting against malformation.

It is therefore important to take account of abortions and stillbirth whereupon the denominator of the rates would be the number of conceptions and not the number of births.

A study of this kind was carried out in New York City between and 1955 (Greenberg, Pelliteri and Barton 1957). As notification of rul

Table 2. *Incidence of abortions and prevalence of malformations at birth in children of mothers who had rubella during pregnancy, according to the stage of pregnancy at the time rubella was contracted (Source: Greenberg, Pelliteri and Barton 1957)*

| | Stage of pregnancy when rubella contracted | | | | | | | |
| | 1st three months | | 2nd three months | | 3rd three months | | Total | |
	No.	(%)	No.	(%)	No.	(%)	No.	(%)
Birth of a normal child	28	(26.9)	74	(83.2)	37	(90.3)	139	(59.4)
Defective child	3	(2.9)	1	(1.1)	0	(0.0)	4	(1.7)
Stillborn	3	(2.9)	2	(2.2)	1	(2.4)	6	(2.6)
Spontaneous abortion	12	(11.5)	1	(1.1)	0	(0.0)	13	(5.6)
Therapeutic abortion (including	48	(46.2)	4	(4.5)	0	(0.0)	52	(22.2)
those for rubella)	(45)		(4)				(49)	
Lost from the study	10	(9.6)	7	(7.9)	3	(7.3)	20	(8.5)
Total	104	(100.0)	89	(100.0)	41	(100.0)	234	(100.0)

was compulsory, all women aged 15–45 years reported as having contracted the disease were asked if they were pregnant. During this seven-year period 24 825 cases of rubella were reported, 2528 of them among women aged 15–45 years; 233 of these women were pregnant and of these 103 were three months pregnant, 86 six months pregnant and 41 in the last three months of pregnancy. The results of this study are shown in Table 2.

The risk of malformation in this population is 2.9 per cent where rubella was contracted during the first three months of pregnancy, i.e. considerably lower than the rates observed in other studies; this is because the rates are based on the number of conceptions rather than the number of births. These conceptions include a considerable number of women who were lost from the study (9.6 per cent) or who had a therapeutic abortion (46.2 per cent of the women exposed to the disease). The proportion of fetuses which would have been born defective and the proportion of normal fetuses in these two groups are unknown.

To compare these rates a control sample of children born to mothers who did not have rubella during pregnancy is required but this is costly

and time-consuming to achieve. While it is relatively easy to follow up and question people if one has a definite reason (e.g. rubella, malformation), it is more difficult to collect a large number of controls. For this, data collected routinely by the health services would be useful—notifications of rubella and notifications of malformation at birth. Cross-checking of these histories would then enable the risks to be calculated. Unfortunately notification of infectious diseases is often regarded as unsatisfactory: even where a system exists registration of malformations at birth is often not carried out. Data relating to abortions are incomplete and are rarely available for earlier than the sixteenth week of pregnancy. As for cross-checking the data, this would be impossible to achieve in many countries where there is no single file in which the entire medical history of patients can be collected so that the pattern of their health from birth to death can be followed.

The prevalence of anomalies at birth may vary according to whether anomalies in induced abortions are included or not. This is important when, for instance in a register of congenital malformations, a comparison of the prevalence of certain malformations at birth in different populations is required, and where the frequency of the practice of abortion varies in proportions often unknown.

The results will also vary with twin births, the malformation criteria and the length of postnatal follow-up. In the study by Greenberg, Pelliteri and Barton (1957) considering twins as a single pregnancy instead of two brings down the rate at birth from 9.7 per cent to 6.4 per cent.

The period of postnatal observation is also important as certain malformations, in particular those characterized by auditory defects, cannot be detected until some time after birth. Prospective studies (Jackson and Fish 1958) have shown that about three-quarters of cases of deafness attributed to rubella may remain undetected up to the age of four years.

PUBLIC HEALTH AND DETERMINATION OF PRIORITIES

The example of rubella illustrates the fundamental importance of an indicator for decisions on health priorities. While a disease may be mild in relation to mortality and morbidity, it could later prove to be of major importance if a relationship is established with an appropriate indicator which in the case of rubella is congenital malformations.

Even if the risk of congenital malformation is lower than was thought at first and is mainly concentrated in the first weeks of pregnancy, the number of non-immunized women exposed to rubella during epidemics makes it a formidable public health problem. The 1964 epidemic on the North American continent is said to have produced 20000 defective children with one or other of the following malformations: ophthalmic lesions such as cataract and glaucoma, deafness, cardiac malformations, lesions of the central nervous system and mental retardation (Rawls et al 1967).

Having been recognized as a major health problem there are two possible preventive actions: the best is of course primary prevention by vaccination; alternatively there is secondary prevention by induced abortion.

EVALUATION OF THE EFFICACY OF VACCINATION
The isolation of the rubella virus, achieved in 1962 using tissue cultures, cleared the path to development of an attenuated live vaccine. Several strains of vaccines were employed (two vaccines are derived from the same strain of HPV-77 virus one of which is produced on duck embryo and the other on dog kidney; a third is prepared from tissue cultures of the Cendehill strain on rabbit kidney; and a fourth is cultured on human diploid cells). Development of a live vaccine gives rise to a number of problems. Traditionally a vaccine must satisfy the following criteria:

it must ensure satisfactory and long-lasting immunity; it must not cause side-effects in the vaccinated person; and it must not cause the virus to be transmitted to associates of the vaccinated person.

As far as rubella is concerned, the sole aim is to prevent the appearance of congenital malformations, i.e. to prevent pregnant women from becoming infected. This raises additional problems such as:

the optimum age for vaccination with regard to duration of immunity;

the risk, which may not be apparent, of reinfection of those vaccinated.

Epidemiological techniques have helped solve some of these problems.

The effectiveness of vaccination must be assessed by serological and epidemiological methods. Serological studies have shown that vaccination gives rise to antibodies in 85–95 per cent of receptive vaccinated patients (Cooper, Giles and Krugman 1963) but titres of antibodies obtained by vaccination are on the whole distinctly lower than the titres obtained after rubella infection (Meyer et al 1969). It is important to know whether those vaccinated really are protected and for how long. Furthermore, while reinfection is unusual after rubella contracted

Table 3. *Rubella attack rate according to age and immunization, Grand Isle, Louisiana, 1970–1971 (Source: Center for Disease Control 1971)*

Age group (years)	Immunized children			Non-immunized children		
	Total	Rubella cases	%	Total	Rubella cases	%
1–10	124	3	2.4	74	16	21.6
11–20	2	0	0	232	75	32.3

naturally, the possibility of reinfection after immunization, perhaps without visible clinical symptoms, must be considered.

A longitudinal study of vaccinated patients and non-vaccinated controls similarly exposed to the virus is the method of choice for assessing the efficacy of vaccination and measuring the degree of protection conferred. This method, which involves the technique of randomized controlled trials, introduces difficult problems both of organization, and in an ethical sense: it is not always possible to use this method.

The efficacy of vaccination can sometimes be estimated from observations made among communities which, because of chance circumstances, reproduce to some extent the conditions of a natural experiment. The 1970–1971 epidemic of Grand Isle, an island near the coast of Louisiana, USA, provides an example (Center for Disease Control 1971). In this community of 2236 inhabitants, 63 per cent of the children aged between one and 10 years, had been vaccinated in an anti-rubella vaccination campaign conducted in August 1970. A few months later when a rubella epidemic broke out (108 cases) the attack rate among non-vaccinated children of up to 10 years of age was found to be nine times higher than in vaccinated children of the same age group. In the older, non-vaccinated children the attack rate was 12 times higher (Table 3). The efficacy of the vaccination is expressed in the following way:

$$\frac{\text{Attack rate among those vaccinated} - \text{Attack rate among those not vaccinated}}{\text{Attack rate among those not vaccinated}}$$

i.e. 92 per cent for the population of Grand Isle under 20 years of age.

By using such carefully analysed observations, repeated in different circumstances, it is possible to assess the efficacy of the vaccination to a satisfactory degree of probability. They are not a substitute for randomized controlled trials. And, of necessity they are belated, whereas vaccination activities were all performed at approximately the same time therefore such analyses can only provide a posteriori information. Also, in order to locate and analyse such epidemics there must be a close and reliable network of epidemiological surveillance.

Interesting data can also be obtained by comparing neighbouring geographical areas assumed to be comparable as far as the epidemiological context is concerned but where the measures employed are different. In the USA, in 1972, a 60.5 per cent decrease was observed in the incidence of rubella in 12 States which had vaccinated over 52 per cent of children in the 1–12 year age group, in contrast with a 49 per cent increase of incidence in States which had vaccinated less than 44 per cent of children in this age group (Center for Disease Control 1971).

INDIVIDUAL PROTECTION AND PROTECTION OF THE COMMUNITY

It is vital not to confuse protection of the individual with protection of a population. Standard epidemiological analysis, either retrospective or prospective, enables comparison of groups of individuals according to whether they have or have not been vaccinated: it provides information on the prophylactic value of a vaccine for the protection of individuals. It does not show what vaccination cover is necessary to prevent the movement of the virus and to protect populations. In the former it is a question of comparing the degree of protection conferred on vaccinated versus non-vaccinated people. In the latter, it is a question of comparing the degree of protection conferred on vaccinated versus non-vaccinated populations.

This distinction, which is sometimes neglected, underlies the frequent confusion found in arguments about the value of massive vaccination of children compared with selective vaccination of women of child-bearing age. These two activities have totally different meanings. Selective vaccination of young women is an individual prophylactic measure, the efficacy and dangers of which are known. Massive vaccination of children is a control measure: it presupposes that young children are the principal source of infection in women of child-bearing age. It therefore aims at reducing the pregnant woman's risk of exposure by reducing the virus reservoir in children. However, it has not yet been possible to measure the efficacy of this method.

While it would rarely be possible to assemble populations subjected to one or the other of these control measures in order to compare them by means of the standard methods of epidemiological analysis, chance observations can again provide valuable information. The Casper epidemic is an example (Klock and Rachelefsky 1973). In this particular district of Wyoming, USA, over 1000 cases of rubella were registered during the first five months of 1971—84 per cent in adolescents of between 12 and 18 years of age. Nine months previously, 83 per cent of children attending primary schools and 52 per cent of those of pre-school age had been vaccinated. It therefore appeared that this vaccination cover of children was not sufficient to control the spread of the disease at least under the conditions prevailing in that district.

This again emphasizes the importance of having available a system of epidemiological surveillance which can collect relevant information and make use of it.

ATTACK RATES AMONG THE CONTACTS OF THOSE VACCINATED

An example of systematic application of the longitudinal approach is provided by study of the dissemination of the virus among associates of people who have been vaccinated. This matter received attention as soon as an anti-rubella vaccine was developed. With natural infection, the virus is present in the nasopharynx. However, as a result of vaccination carried out in pregnant women and followed by abortion, it is known that the infection of such women by the attenuated virus can be transmitted to the fetus (Modlin et al 1976). It is therefore vital to ensure that the attenuated virus cannot be transmitted to other people, as this could constitute a hazard for pregnant women coming into contact with people who have been vaccinated.

To solve this problem, over a period of 24 months (1970–1972) 11 635 women admitted for confinement or abortion to four hospitals in Nashville, Tennessee, were questioned about their history of contacts with vaccinated persons during the first three months of pregnancy or the three months prior to conception (Fleet et al 1975). The definition of contact was precise, close contact being taken as the fact of having been close (5 m at most) to a vaccinated person for at least one minute on enclosed premises. It was possible to reconstitute the histories of 10 010 women; 989 were classified as contacts with vaccinated persons and 9021 as non-contacts. Furthermore, for 3990 women, there were results available of paired serological tests taken at the beginning of and during pregnancy. The incidence of sero-conversion and abortion were compared for women who had had contact with vaccinated persons and those who had not, as was the proportion of aborted fetuses in which the rubella virus was

Table 4. *Complications of pregnancy and anomalies in the newborn child according to the contact antecedents during pregnancy with persons vaccinated against rubella (Source: Fleet et al 1975)*

Exposure	Number	Congenital rubella syndrome	Anomalies associated with rubella	Abortions
Contact with vaccinated persons	989	0 (0%)	0 (0%)	16 (1.62%)
No contact with vaccinated persons	9021	8 (0.9%)	28 (0.31%)	92 (1.02%)

recovered, and the prevalence at birth of congenital anomalies associated with rubella and of anomalies compatible with the congenital rubella syndrome (hepatosplenomegaly and purpura with thrombocytopaenia).

The haemagglutination levels were found to be similar in the two groups. Except for abortions, which were significantly more frequent in the contacts, no differences were noted in relation to the development of pregnancy. It was therefore concluded that vaccination with attenuated live virus was harmless for women associated with those who had been vaccinated.

SECONDARY PREVENTION: DEFINITION OF VULNERABLE GROUPS

In many countries rubella in mothers at the beginning of pregnancy constitutes an indication for induced abortion, but one has to distinguish the risks. It may be a case of either, clinically diagnosed rubella; serologically confirmed rubella in a susceptible woman; inadvertent vaccination of a pregnant woman (with risk altered by the stage of pregnancy); contact with someone who had rubella; or pregnancy during an epidemic. The risk will vary considerably with the specificity of the criterion employed.

Longitudinal studies have shown that approximately 30 per cent of the women who present clinically diagnosed rubella during the first month of pregnancy and whose pregnancy reaches full term give birth to malformed children. The risk is higher if the infection has been confirmed serologically, thus excluding risks of error in diagnosis of the rash.

The risk from contact with a rubella case is lower. It presupposes that the exposure of a sero-negative woman has led to infection, which may not be apparent. The studies carried out at Nashville (Fleet et al 1975) revealed two cases of congenital anomalies or the syndrome compatible with congenital rubella (0.76 per cent) among 266 mothers who had been in contact with rubella during the first three months of pregnancy or during the three months prior to conception compared with 36 cases (0.33 per cent) in 10 888 mothers who had no such contact.

As for the risk associated with pregnancy during an epidemic, this brings in a number of probabilities including the risk of infection which in its turn depends on the attack rate in the population and also on the chance that the exposed woman may be sero-negative and therefore susceptible.

By means of epidemiological studies it is possible to determine the risk of malformation at birth as well as the risk of removing a normal product of conception, depending on the sensitivity and specificity of the criteria employed. Such studies thus help to provide the elements necessary for a decision on abortion.

REFERENCES

Bradford Hill, A., Doll, R., McL. Galloway, T. & Hughes, J. P. W. (1958) Virus diseases in pregnancy and congenital defects. *British Journal of Preventive and Social Medicine, 12,* 1

Center for Disease Control (1971) *Rubella Surveillance.* USPHS, Atlanta, Georgia (October) *3,* 15

Cooper, L. Z., Giles, J. P. & Krugman, S. (1963) Clinical trial of live attenuated rubella virus vaccine, HPV-77 strain. *American Journal of Diseases of Children, 115,* 655

Fleet, W. F., Vaughn, W., Lefkowitz, L. B., Schaffner, W., Federspiel, C. F., Thompson, J. & Karzon, D. T. (1975) Gestational exposure to rubella vaccines. A population surveillance study. *American Journal of Epidemiology, 101,* 220

Greenberg, M., Pelliteri, O. & Barton, J. (1957) Frequency of defects in infants whose mothers had rubella during pregnancy. *Journal of the American Medical Association, 165,* 675

Gregg, N. M. (1941) Congenital cataract following German measles in the mother. *Transactions of the Ophthalmological Society of Australia, 3,* 35

Ingalls, T. M., Sabbott, F. L., Hampson, K. W. & Gordon, J. E. (1960) Rubella: its epidemiology and teratology. In *Preventive Medicine and Epidemiology.* Gordon, J. E. & Ingalls, T. H. (eds). *American Journal of Medical Sciences, 239,* 363

Jackson, A. D. M. & Fish, L. (1958) Deafness following maternal rubella; results of a prospective investigation. *Lancet, 2,* 1241

Klock, L. E. & Rachelefsky, G. S. (1973) Failure of rubella herd immunity during an epidemic. *New England Journal of Medicine, 238,* 69

Lundström, R. (1952) Rubella during pregnancy. Its effects upon perinatal mortality, the incidence of congenital abnormalities and immaturity. A preliminary report. *Acta Paediatrica, 41,* 583

Meyer, H. M., Jr., Parkman, P. D., Horbins, T. E., Larson, M. E., Davis, W. J., Simsarian, J. P. & Hopps, H. E. (1969) Attenuated rubella viruses laboratory and clinical characteristics. *American Journal of Diseases of Children, 118,* 155

Modlin, J. F., Herrmann, K., Brandling-Bennett, A. D., Eddings, D. L. & Hayden, G. F. (1976) Risk of congenital abnormality after inadvertent rubella vaccination of pregnant women. *New England Journal of Medicine, 294,* 972

Rawls, W. E., Melnick, J. L., Bradstreet, C. M. P., Bailey, M., Ferris, A. A., Lehmann, N. J., Nagler, F. P., Furesz, J., Kono, R., Ohtawara, M., Halonen, P., Stewart, J., Ryan, J. M., Strauss, J., Zdnazilek, J., Leerhoy, J., von Magnus, H., Sohier, R. & Ferreira, W. (1967) WHO collaborative study on the sero-epidemiology of rubella. *Bulletin of the World Health Organization, 37,* 79

Swan, C., Tostevin, A. L., Mayo, H. & Black, G. M. B. (1943) Congenital defects in infants following infectious diseases during pregnancy, with special reference to relationship between German measles and cataract, deaf-mutism, heart disease and microcephaly, and to period of pregnancy in which occurrence of rubella is followed by congenital abnormalities. *Medical Journal of Australia, 2,* 201

Warkany, J. & Kalter, H. (1961) Congenital malformations. *New England Journal of Medicine, 265,* 993

Wesselhoeft, C. (1949) Rubella (German measles) and congenital deformities. *New England Journal of Medicine, 240,* 258

SUGGESTED TEXTS FOR BACKGROUND READING

Alderson, M. (1976) *An Introduction to Epidemiology.* London: Macmillan. p 226

Barker, D. J. P. & Rose, G. (1976) *Epidemiology in Medical Practice.* Edinburgh: Churchill Livingstone. p 140

Barker, D. J. P. & Bennet, F. J. (1976) *Practical Epidemiology* (2nd ed) Edinburgh: Churchill Livingstone. p 180

Jenicek, M. (1976) *Introduction à l'Epidémiologie.* Quebec & Paris: Edisem & Maloine

Lilienfeld, A. M. (1976) *Foundations of Epidemiology.* New York: Oxford University Press

MacMahon, B. & Pugh, T. F. (1970) *Epidemiology: Principles and Methods.* Boston: Little Brown

Mausner, J. S. & Bahn, A. K. (1974) *Epidemiology—An Introductory Text.* Philadelphia: W. B. Saunders. p 377

Morris, J. N. (1975) *Uses of Epidemiology.* (Third edition) London: Churchill Livingstone

Rumeau-Rouquette, C. & Schwartz, D. (1970) *Méthodes en Epidémiologie.* Paris: Flammarion. p 272

CHAPTER 16

Causation and Control with Special Reference to Cigarette Smoking

Louis Massé and Geneviève Massé

This chapter describes the use of epidemiological methods in determining the chronic health effects of smoking. Detailed descriptions of a number of well known retrospective and prospective studies of the relationship between lung cancer and smoking are given including Doll and Hill's study of British Doctors. These are followed by information about experimental studies of carcinogenesis in animals.

Some ideas about why people take up smoking are followed by discussion of the possible ways of reducing the damage done to health and of the need for effective ways of dissuading people from taking up the habit.

The following illustration of the application and development of knowledge of the health effects of smoking by epidemiological study compliments Lechat's description of development of knowledge of rubella in Chapter 15. The application of epidemiological methods to smoking has been chosen to demonstrate how the methods used for infectious diseases are applied to chronic non-infectious diseases and human behaviour.

HISTORY OF SMOKING AND KNOWLEDGE OF ITS HEALTH EFFECTS

Tobacco was introduced by explorers from the New World into Spain and England in the sixteenth century and argument soon developed about the effect on humans of use, by combustion or other means, of the leaf and its products. While pipe smoking, chewing or 'snuffing' tobacco were reputed to be pleasurable and even of medicinal value (it also created considerable tax revenue!), smoking was also condemned as a 'foul smelling and loathsome custom' harmful to the brain and lungs. The major question of whether smoking was good or bad for health thus remained until early this century when scientists began to take an interest in the health effects of tobacco. Only in the last three decades have definitive epidemiological studies been undertaken on the health effects of smoking.

The data of vital statisticians in the early 1900s are normally taken to be the starting point of studies into the relationship between smoking and other tobacco usage and lung cancer, other cancers, diseases of the circulatory system and non-cancerous conditions of the respiratory tract, e.g. chronic bronchitis.

Around 1930 conspicuous increases in mortality incidence from these causes became apparent and resulted in a number of investigations and the setting up of various governmental committees to study the association between smoking and health. However it was not until 30 years later that the Advisory Committee of the Surgeon General in the US Public Health Service published its notable report entitled *Smoking and Health* (US Department of Health, Education and Welfare, 1964). This covered the criteria for epidemiological methods for use in relevant studies. It stated:

'In carrying out the studies through the use of this epidemiologic method, many factors, variables and results or investigations must be considered to determine first whether an association actually exists between an attribute or agent and a disease. Judgement on this point is based upon indirect and direct measures of the suggested association. If it be shown that an association exists, then the question is asked: "Does the association have a causal significance?"

'Statistical methods cannot establish proof of a causal relationship in an association. The causal significance of an association is a matter of judgement which goes beyond any statement of statistical probability. To judge or evaluate the causal significance of the association between the attribute or agent and the disease, or effect upon health, a number of criteria must be utilized, no one of which is an all-sufficient basis for judgement. These criteria include:

'(a) The consistency of the association
(b) The strength of the association
(c) The specificity of the association
(d) The temporal relationship of the association
(e) The coherence of the association.'

RETROSPECTIVE STUDIES

These are usually designed to establish if a particular attribute is associated with a disease. In practice a group of patients with a particular disease is compared to a group of controls with regard to the frequency of the suspect attribute. Significant differences may be found which will lead to agreement about association but this does not provide any idea of the difference in the relative risk of suffering from the disease in those with and without the attribute.

Chapter 5 by Rumeau-Rouquette details the methods of determining relative risk, the problems of interpretation and the prerequisites for undertaking retrospective studies. These methods have been used by a number of investigators to study the relationships between smoking and lung cancer.

Studies by Doll and Hill (1950) and Wynder and Graham (1950) are good early examples of the use of the retrospective study technique and many others have followed their example. Doll and Hill (1950) used two separate control groups: the first were patients suffering from conditions other than cancer who were matched with lung cancer patients in four respects—sex, five-year age groups, being inpatients in the same hospital, and there at about the same time; the second group were patients suffering from cancer of the stomach, colon or rectum but these patients were not matched with the lung cancer patients as were the first non-cancer group although their presence in the hospital was notified in the same way as for the lung cancer patients.

It was hoped that by notifying all cancer patients in the same way without specifying the site of the primary tumour investigators could interview these patients about their smoking habits without introducing subconscious bias by the interviewers knowing to which group the patients belonged.

This second control group served three purposes. These were: to test if any differences found between lung cancer patients and matched controls were characteristic of only lung cancer or of cancer generally; to test whether the differences found could be because of a personal element in the choice of controls or whether these differences were also found if controls were chosen independently of the investigators; thirdly, it was hoped to be able to test whether differences arose because of bias by the interviewer as a result of knowing in which group a patient was. But this aim was not fulfilled because the interviewer eventually became aware of most diagnoses. The study showed a marked difference in the smoking habits of patients with lung cancer and those with other diseases: the former were more likely to smoke and also smoked more heavily than the latter.

Schwartz and Denoix (1957) performed a similar study in France using four separate control groups all matched with lung cancer patients for age and sex, for hospitals in which patients were treated, for time of interview and for the person who did the interviewing. The four groups were:

1. patients with cancer elsewhere in the upper respiratory or digestive tract;
2. patients with other types of primary cancer;
3. patients with non-cancerous diseases;
4. patients admitted with traffic or occupational injuries.

No significant differences were found in the smoking habits of men in groups 2, 3 and 4, but a sharp difference was found between these three groups and the lung cancer patients. Men in category 1 occupied an intermediate position with respect to smoking habits.

Such studies are however open to criticism because there are several ways in which bias might have been introduced. It is possible in Doll and Hill's investigation (1950) that patient or interviewer overestimated the amount smoked because either might have suspected the diagnosis (although interviewers were not actually informed of the diagnosis). However the findings in a small group who were wrongly diagnosed as having lung cancer negate this criticism. At the time of the interview they were thought to be suffering from lung cancer but their smoking habits were found to be in line with the control group rather than with those of confirmed lung cancer patients.

Another criticism is that a control group of other patients in the same hospital might not be representative of the smoking habits in the population from which they come. Comparison of hospital control groups who normally live in the Greater London area with groups in the general population show that the hospital controls actually smoke more. This might be expected in view of the association of smoking with a number of other diseases. But if anything this would tend to lead to an underestimation of the effects of smoking in predisposing to lung cancer.

These and other studies have led to a calculation of a relative risk among smokers of developing lung cancer of between 5 and 14 fold in excess of the risk in non-smokers. This risk increases with the amount smoked. In *Smoking and Health* (USDHEW 1964) it was stated:

'In retrospective studies, the smoking histories of persons with a specified disease (for example lung cancer), are compared with those of appropriate control groups without the disease. For lung cancer alone, 29 such retrospective studies have been made in recent years. Despite many variations in design and method, all but one (which dealt with females) showed that proportionately more cigarette smokers are found among the lung cancer patients than in the control populations without lung cancer.

'Extensive retrospective studies of the prevalence of specific symptoms and signs—chronic cough, sputum production, breathlessness, chest illness and decreased lung function consistently show that these occur more often in cigarette smokers than in non-smokers. Some of these signs and symptoms are the clinical expressions of chronic bronchitis and some are associated more with emphysema; in general, they increase with amount of smoking and decrease after cessation of smoking.'

As mentioned earlier the objective of a retrospective study is to determine the frequency of a particular attribute among cases and controls, but to make estimates of the relative risk of developing the disease in question certain assumptions have to be made—and these are often somewhat suspect which is when prospective studies become useful.

PROSPECTIVE STUDIES

These have been used to determine the risk of developing various diseases as a result of smoking. Doll and Hill (1954) began the first prospective study of general and cause specific mortality among British doctors. Questionnaires were sent to all men and women on the British Medical Register, out of 59 600 doctors useful replies were sent back by 41 000. Information was gathered on whether each doctor was a smoker, an ex-smoker or had never smoked; at what age each smoker took up the habit; and the method and quantity of smoking. Ex-smokers gave information about when they gave up the habit and they all had to state their age and address.

Two 10-year follow-up surveys have taken place (Doll and Hill 1964; Doll and Peto 1976). The Registrars General provided information on the majority of deaths where the recorded occupation showed the subject to be medically qualified. In the case of those who could not be recorded in this way, for example army officers, university teachers or dentists, or those who died abroad the information on deaths was obtained from the General Medical Council or the British Medical Association. Information on nearly every death was obtained.

The most recent analysis of this study (Doll and Peto 1976) shows that increased mortality risk from lung cancer in males was: about seven fold for those smoking 10 cigarettes a day; 13 fold for those smoking 20 cigarettes a day; and 25 fold for those smoking 30 cigarettes a day.

Hammond and Horn (1954; 1958 a and b) obtained similar information using a different technique. With the sponsorship of the American Cancer Society 22 000 members (volunteers) were asked to record the smoking histories of 10 male acquaintances aged 50–69 years, not at the time known to be seriously ill, and with whom the volunteers expected to remain in contact. The volunteers then reported at annual intervals whether their acquaintances were still alive. About 190 000 completed forms were received initially: 44 months later 92.7 per cent were reported to be still alive, 6.2 per cent (11 870) had died and 1.1 per cent (2071) had been lost to follow-up. The mortality by different causes could be calculated and, as for Doll and Hill's study, comparison of mortality by smoking category could be made. The death rates from lung cancer per 1000 men per year were as follows: 0.13 for non-smokers; 0.95 for those smoking 1–9 cigarettes a day; 1.08 for those smoking 10–20 cigarettes a day; 2.29 for those smoking 21–40 cigarettes a day; and 2.64 for those smoking 41 +; i.e. the excess risk for those smoking 21–40 cigarettes every day was 17.6 and 20.3 for those smoking more.

These major prospective studies of lung cancer mortality have also shown that the risk decreases in those who stop smoking; this decreased risk becomes apparent within a few years. Also in smokers the risk increases with age but in ex-smokers the risk stays constant. After 10 years risk for the ex-smoker is about a quarter of what it is for men of the same age who continue to smoke.

Doll and Peto's study (1976) probably gives the best illustration of the effect on lung cancer mortality of stopping smoking. Over 50 per cent of the doctors who smoked at the start of the 20 year study in 1954 had stopped by 1971. These data on doctors' smoking enabled a comparison with the general population of England and Wales where fewer people have given up, in terms of lung cancer mortality over the period 1954–1971. In all men under 65 years old the lung cancer mortality rate rose slightly while in doctors over the same period it fell by a total of 40 per cent (Figure 1). For those aged 65 years and over, again lung cancer mortality in the general male population rose markedly but the rate for doctors fell and then rose again slightly. Lower initial levels in doctors shown in Figure 1 may be because of sample selection or because a smaller proportion of doctors actually smokes or because they tend to start smoking later in life compared to other men.

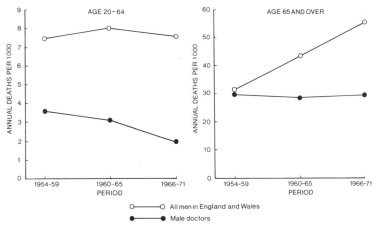

Figure 1. Death rates from lung cancer in British male doctors and in all men in England and Wales 1954–1971 (Source: Doll & Peto 1976 in Royal College of Physicians 1977)

EXPERIMENTAL STUDIES

Several hundred compounds have been isolated from the tobacco leaf including cellulose products, proteins, starches, sugars, alkaloids, pectin substances, hydrocarbons, phenols, fatty acids, isoprenoids, sterols and various inorganic minerals.

Smoke from tobacco is a mixture of 300 compounds either in the gaseous form or as minute droplets ranging from 10 to 40 millionths of an inch in diameter. The exact composition varies with type of tobacco, method of curing and the way it is smoked. About 50 per cent of inhaled smoke is retained in the lungs; some droplets are deposited on the walls of the bronchial tract while others are taken up by motile cells mainly in the air sacs.

The smoke produced by cigarettes is faintly acid in contrast to the slightly alkaline smoke of pipes or cigars. It is because alkaline smoke is more irritating that cigarette smoke is more readily inhaled.

The types of compound in tobacco smoke which are of interest medically are:

1 Nicotine
Up to 3 mg of nicotine can be recovered from the smoke of one cigarette. The amount absorbed ranges from 90 per cent to 10 per cent depending on inhalation habits. A recent study has compared the nicotine in the

blood stream of cigarette smokers with the level in those who smoke other tobacco products (Turner, Sillett and McNicol 1977).

2 *Carcinogenic substances*
So far 16 substances capable of initiating cancer in experimental animals have been identified in tobacco smoke, most in minute amounts. Skin cancer can be produced in mice by application of tar condensed from tobacco smoke and some animals develop lung cancer if exposed to tobacco smoke in inhaled air.

3 *Irritants*
A number of substances are present in tobacco smoke which affect the mucous membrane, chiefly in the respiratory tract, by stimulating excess secretion of mucus and delaying its removal by slowing the action of the ciliated bronchial tube lining. Substances producing this effect include ammonia, volatile acids, aldehydes, phenols and ketones.

4 *Carbon monoxide*
In heavy smokers the proportion of haemoglobin in the blood combined with carbon monoxide instead of oxygen (thus reducing the oxygen carrying efficiency of the blood) is about 5 per cent but it may rise to over 10 per cent when a number of cigarettes are smoked in succession. It is thought by some to play a role in the aetiology of coronary heart disease.

5 *Arsenic*
The presence of this substance in cigarettes is caused by the use of arsenic-containing insecticides but this has declined and the quantity of arsenic found in cigarettes is now minute. Although it has never been present in sufficient quantities to cause cancer on its own it might have had an aggravant or co-carcinogenic action which cannot be dismissed.

Some more details about animal experiments are of interest here. Some animal species have such efficient nasal filtering systems that little smoke reaches their lungs; other species, however, have been used to demonstrate severe pathological changes in the respiratory tract after long exposure to cigarette smoke.

Dontenwill et al (1973) have shown that Syrian golden hamsters develop severe changes in the cells lining the larynx and early evasive cancer if they are exposed to cigarette smoke in their lifetime: these changes varied with the particular strain of the hamster species studies (Bernfeld, Homburger and Russfield 1974).

Rats exposed to cigarette smoke in their lifetime show changes in the lining cells of the lungs which pathologists believe is a stage in development of cancer (Davis et al 1975).

Auerbach et al (1970) showed that dogs exposed to cigarette smoke through an artificial opening in the windpipe develop more tumours than those not exposed. However, in only two of the dogs studied were the tumours similar to smoking-related human cancers.

Finally Harris et al (1974) showed that mice who breathe a mixture of cigarette smoke and air at short, frequent intervals are more likely to develop cancers than control animals.

SMOKING—A PRIORITY PROBLEM

Observations on smoking and lung cancer have led to a number of epidemiological surveys of other health consequences of smoking. As a result, it has been shown that smoking is associated with a number of other diseases. Fletcher and Horn (1970) listed the relative risk of dying from various causes as follows:

Causes of death	Relative risk smokers/ non- smokers	Causes of death	Relative risk smokers/ non- smokers
Cancer of the lung	10.8	Cirrhosis of the liver	2.2
Bronchitis and emphysema	6.1	Cancer of bladder	1.9
Cancer of larynx	5.4	Coronary artery diseases	1.7
Cancer of oral cavity	4.1	Other heart diseases	1.7
Cancer of oesophagus	3.4	Hypertensive heart diseases	1.5
Stomach and duodenal ulcers	2.8	General arteriosclerosis	1.5
Circulatory diseases	2.6	Cancer of kidney	1.5

Until about 20 years ago it was thought that smoking harmed only those with certain uncommon diseases, but it is now recognised that smokers are particularly prone to disabling and fatal diseases and as a result non-smokers are likely to be more healthy and to live longer than smokers.

Prospective studies of death rates among smokers have enabled calculation of the years of life a smoker may forfeit according to the number of cigarettes smoked and also the loss of expectation of life per cigarette smoked. Using data from Doll and Peto (1976) it can be calculated that a smoker of 20 cigarettes a day can expect to live five years less than he might have done if he were a non-smoker.

Cigarette smoking may also cause prolonged ill health. An individual may sustain repeated heart attacks and may well be chronically disabled as a result and the sufferer from chronic bronchitis may suffer 10 years of being severely short of breath before death.

Chronic disabling conditions are not the only effects of cigarette smoking: cigarette smokers are also more prone to attacks of acute bronchitis and other chest illnesses. It has been calculated that 50 million working days are lost every year in industry in the United Kingdom as a result of cigarette smoking. Smith (1972) has shown that people who smoke more than 20 cigarettes a day have twice as many days off work as non-smokers.

We have concentrated on the contribution that retrospective and prospective studies have made to improving the evidence for a relationship between smoking and disease, especially lung cancer. However, the major role of vital statistics should not be forgotten. This contribution which led to further investigations is well recorded in the first report to the US Surgeon General (USDHEW 1964) and *Smoking and Health* from the UK Royal College of Physicians (1962). Prevalence studies have also made a major contribution in increasing knowledge about smoking and its association with chronic bronchitis.

PREVALENCE STUDIES

Interest in chronic bronchitis increased following the famous London smog of 1952. An example of the methods used to elucidate the relationship between smoking and chronic bronchitis can be described as follows: individuals with the same occupation, but living in rural or urban areas, were investigated using standard questionnaires and standard tests of ventilatory function. It was found that symptom level and ventilatory function were associated with area of residence and smoking habits but it was also found that smoking was most closely associated with symptom level and ventilatory function independent of area of residence (Holland and Reid 1965; Holland et al 1965).

Similar studies have been done in relation to coronary heart disease, but, as has been shown earlier in this chapter, lung cancer sufferers are relatively uncommon and are unlikely to live long with the disease so it is not suitable for prevalence studies.

PREVENTION

Having established the importance of smoking as a health problem it is now worth considering what could be done to reduce its effects by various levels of preventive activity.

Like other forms of drug dependence smoking is a habit which is easily acquired but difficult to give up. *Smoking or Health* (Roy. Coll. Phys 1977) describes the various theories proposed for why people take up smoking. The headings may appear a little artificial because they are often interrelated.

'*Genetic*. It has been claimed that genetic factors may determine smoking behaviour, and that cancer-proneness, extraversion, a pyknic build, and a tendency to smoke are inherited together. Studies of twins provide some evidence of a genetic influence in that identical twins, even if reared apart, are more similar in their smoking habits than are non-identical twins. In general, however, inheritance appears to be less important than environment in determining smoking behaviour.

'*Personality*. Many workers have attempted to identify a "smoking type" of personality, but the distinctions between the personalities of smokers and non-smokers are small.

'*Social*. Several investigations have brought out a fairly consistent pattern of important social factors. These are by far the dominating influence in starting to smoke and second only to pharmacological factors in maintaining the habit. Social class, example and precept from parents and older siblings, type of school and age of leaving school are all strong influences. Perhaps the most powerful determinant is the number of friends who smoke.

'*Psychodynamic*. The two most plausible theories suggest that smoking is a compensatory activity for early oral deprivation, or for underlying sense of inferiority.' (N.B. Despite quotation of this passage this is now widely disbelieved.)

'*Sensorimotor*. For some smokers it is the smoking act itself that forms the basis of the habit rather than psychosocial or pharmacological effects.' (Again there is little evidence for this theory.)

'*Pharmacological*. Cigarette smoking allows the absorption of about 0.05 to 0.15 mg nicotine per puff.' (Heavy smokers are in fact dependent on nicotine and actually require a regular 'fix' to prevent the discomfort of withdrawal symptoms.)'

It has been established that social and pharmacological factors are probably the most important in establishing and maintaining the smoking habit and as a result certain actions can be taken to perhaps dissuade people from smoking.

ANTI-SMOKING ACTION BY GOVERNMENT OR OTHER AUTHORITIES

Acceptance by governments of the health dangers of smoking illustrated in so many studies has led to a variety of actions:

1. Increased taxation on cigarettes and other tobacco products.
2. Health warnings on cigarette packets.
3. Banning of television advertising of cigarettes.
4. Government financed counter-advertising.
5. To reduce the health risk and annoyance of passive inhalation of smoke by non-smokers more public areas such as hospital, public transport and entertainment facilities have areas where smoking is prohibited. This health risk of passive smoking has been illustrated in a study by Colley, Holland and Corkhill (1974) who showed that newborn babies exposed to parents' cigarette smoke are twice as likely to develop bronchitis or pneumonia in the first year of life as babies not exposed to parents' cigarette smoke.
6. Introduction of less harmful cigarettes by reduction of tar and nicotine levels, alterations in method used to cure tobacco, and increased efficiency of filters.
7. In some countries cellulose-based materials are being incorporated into some cigarettes as a tobacco replacement.
8. Norway and Sweden have proposed that all children born in 1974 should grow up as non-smokers.

For those who want to give up smoking a variety of clinics, advisory centres, counselling sessions and drug treatment regimens have been introduced but all with little success. Further work is necessary in the development of suitable programmes in this context.

Effective reduction in the health consequences of smoking is a more fruitful field for study. Appropriate methods to discourage children from starting to smoke are required but development of suitable and effective programmes is a major task. A five-year longitudinal study is in progress under the direction of the Department of Community Medicine at St Thomas' Hospital to identify children at risk of becoming smokers and to enable effective educational programmes to be developed (Banks et al 1978).

CONCLUSION

This chapter has highlighted the major contribution made by various types of epidemiological study in determining the hazards of smoking. It is by no means an exhaustive coverage of the subject but a number of publications may be of further use (see Suggested Texts). As well as covering the contribution of research the chapter has attempted to describe the criteria on which such studies should be judged in assessing their impact on health.

Suggestions about preventive action have been made but it is apparent that only primary prevention, i.e. stopping people from ever taking up the habit, will be effective in reducing lung cancer mortality and morbidity and mortality from other smoking-related disease. There is even evidence that screening for lung cancer is ineffective in reducing mortality (Colley 1974).

Hopefully this chapter has given some idea of how the methods described earlier in this book can be applied to development of knowledge on a particular health problem and application of this knowledge to determination of health policy.

REFERENCES

Auerbach, O., Hammond, E. C., Kirman, D., Garfinkel, L. & Stout, A. P. (1967) Histologic changes in bronchial tubes of cigarette smoking dogs. *Cancer* (New York), *20*, 2055

Banks, M. H., Bewley, B. R., Bland, J. M., Dean, J. R., & Pollard, V. (1978) Long-term study of smoking by secondary schoolchildren. *Archives of Disease in Childhood*, *53*, 12

Bernfeld, P., Homburger, F. & Russfield, A. B. (1974) Strain differences in the response of inbred Syrian hamsters to cigarette smoke inhalation. *Journal of the National Cancer Institute*, *53*, 1141

Colley, J. R. T. (1974) Diseases of the lung. Screening for disease (Series) *Lancet* Oct 5–Dec 21.

Colley, J. R., Holland, W. W. & Corkhill, R. T. (1974) Influence of passive smoking and parental phlegm on pneumonia and bronchitis in early childhood. *Lancet*, *2*, 1031.

Davis, B. R., Whitehead, J. K., Gill, M. E., Lee, P. M., Butterworth, A. D. & Roe, F. J. C. (1975) Response of the rat lung to inhaled tobacco smoke with or without prior exposure to 3, 4-benzpyrene (BP) given by intractracheal instillation. *British Journal of Cancer*, *31*, 469

Doll, W. R. & Hill, A. B. (1950) Smoking and carcinoma of the lung *British Medical Journal*, *2*, 739

Doll, W. R. & Hill, A. B. (1954) The mortality of doctors in relation to their smoking habits: a preliminary report. *British Medical Journal*, *1*, 1451

Doll, R. & Hill, A. B. (1964) Mortality in relation to smoking: ten years' observations of British doctors. *British Medical Journal*, *1*, 1399 and 1460

Doll, W. R. & Peto, R. (1976) Mortality in relation to smoking: 20 years' observations on male British doctors. *British Medical Journal*, *2*, 1525

Dontenwill, W., Chevalier, H. J., Harke, H. P., Klimisch, H. J., Reckzeh, G. & Schneider, B. (1973) Investigations on the effects of chronic cigarette-smoke inhalation in Syrian Golden hamsters. *Journal of the National Cancer Institute*, *51*, 1781

Fletcher, C. M. & Horn, D. (1970) Smoking and health. World Health Organization Chronicle, *24*, 345

Hammond, E. C. & Horn, D. (1954) The relationship between human smoking habits and death rates. A follow-up study of 187766 men. *Journal of American Medical Association*, *155*, 1316

Hammond, E. C., & Horn, D. (1958a) Smoking and death rates—report on forty-four months follow-up of 187783 men. I Total mortality. *Journal of the American Medical Association*, *166*, 1159

Hammond, E. C. & Horn, D. (1958b) Smoking and death rates—report on the forty-four months follow-up of 187783 men. II Death rates by cause. *Journal of the American Medical Association*, *166*, 1294

Harris, R. J. C., Negroni, G., Ludgate, S., Pick, G. R., Chesterman, F. C. & Maidment, B. J. (1974) The incidence of lung tumours in C 57 BL mice exposed to cigarette smoke/air mixtures for prolonged periods. *International Journal of Cancer*, *14*, 30

Holland, W. W. & Reid, D. D. (1965) The urban factors in chronic bronchitis. *Lancet*, *1*, 445

Holland, W. W., Reid, D. D., Seltzer, R. & Stone, R. W. (1965) Respiratory disease in England and the United States. Studies of comparative prevalence. *Archives of Environmental Health*, *10*, 338

Royal College of Physicians (1962) *Smoking and Health*. Tunbridge Wells: Pitman Medical.

Royal College of Physicians (1977) *Smoking or Health*. Tunbridge Wells: Pitman Medical.

Smith, D. J. (1972) Absenteeism and ' presenteeism ' in industry. *Archives of Environmental Health*, *21*, 345

Turner, J. A. McM., Sillett, R. W. & McNicol, M. W. (1977) Effect of cigar smoking on carboxyhaemoglobin and plasma nicotine concentrations in primary pipe and cigar smokers and ex-cigarette smokers. *British Medical Journal*, *2*, 1387

US Department of Health Education and Welfare. (1964) *Smoking and Health*. PHS Pub No. 1104, Washington.

Wynder, E. L. & Graham, E. A. (1950) Tobacco smoking as a possible etiologic factor in bronchiogenic carcinoma. A study of six hundred and eighty four proved cases. *Journal of the American Medical Association*, *143*, 329

SUGGESTED TEXTS FOR BACKGROUND READING

Royal College of Physicians (1962) *Smoking and Health*. Tunbridge Wells: Pitman Medical.

The Second World Conference on Smoking and Health (1972) Bath: Pitman Medical.

The Third World Conference on Smoking and Health (1975) New York: USDHEW Pub No. (NIH) 76-1221.

World Conference on Smoking and Health (1968) A summary of the Proceedings. New York: American Cancer Society.

US Department of Health, Education and Welfare (1964) *Smoking and Health*. PHS Pub No. 1103, Washington.

POSTSCRIPT

Postscript

Leo A. Kaprio

It is with great interest that I have read this book. It appears to be not only a new and fascinating piece of reading but also a book which is greatly needed. It has become increasingly important not only in health, but in many other fields, to attempt to gain some kind of perspective before embarking on new, or continuing on old, ventures. The rapid development of new technologies within and outside the health field, the ever-increasing cost of health protection and maintenance, the complexity of contemporary health care and growing aspirations and expectations of people are some of the challenges faced by those responsible for health policy and delivery of health care. To meet these challenges, guidance and support from various disciplines are needed. It is difficult to overemphasize the role that epidemiology has to play in this respect: as a science concerned with occurrence, progression and causation of disease as well as the development of new approaches to prevention and control of modern epidemics of degenerative, neoplastic and traumatic diseases; as a basic tool of planning and management of health services; and finally as a means and method of evaluating the outcome of various health interventions and services.

The World Health Organization has always recognized the importance of the scientific basis of the development of health services. The Sixth General Programme of Work of WHO covering the period 1978–1983 lists among the principal programme objectives the need for the promotion and development of biomedical and health services research. It also calls for the promotion of systems for continued planning, programming and management including evaluation of health promoting activities, since these are the main mechanisms for programme development. Again this book is a very good illustration of what epidemiology and epidemiological research have to offer in achieving these objectives.

There is another aspect of this book I would like to emphasize. On several occasions over the last few years WHO has stressed that the global social goal is the provision of an acceptable level of health care to all

260

members of society and set the year 2000 as a possible target date. It has also been stated that this target could be attained if each Member State were to exercise the political will to reset its health priorities in accordance with their social relevance for the total national population, and at the same time, to participate actively in the international endeavour for global health promotion.

This book is a good example of such an international endeavour being the outcome of cooperation by the Members of the European Community. I hope it will strengthen the penetration of sound health concepts and technologies to serve the populations of all the Member States of the European Region of WHO and also will potentially increase the opportunities for WHO to be useful throughout the world.

INDEX

Index